Systematic Reviews in Health Care
A Practical Guide

What do we do if different clinical studies appear to give different answers? This user-friendly introduction to this difficult subject provides a clear, unintimidating and structured approach to systematic reviews and incorporates several key features:

- A practical guide to meta-analysis and the fundamental basis of evidence-based medicine
- A step-by-step explanation of how to undertake a systematic review and the pitfalls to avoid
- Liberally illustrated with explanatory examples and exercises
- A review of the available software for meta-analysis

Whether applying research to questions for individual patients or for health policy, one of the challenges is interpreting apparently conflicting research. A systematic review is a method of systematically identifying relevant research, appraising its quality and synthesizing the results. The last two decades have seen increasing interest and developments in methods for doing high-quality systematic reviews. Part 1 of this book provides a clear introduction to the concepts of reviewing, and lucidly describes the difficulties and traps to avoid. A unique feature of the book is its description, in Part 2, of the different methods needed for different types of health care questions: frequency of disease, prognosis, diagnosis, risk and management. As well as illustrative examples, there are exercises for each of the sections.

This is essential reading for those interested in synthesizing health care research, and for those studying for a degree in Public Health.

Paul Glasziou is Professor of Evidence-based Medicine in the School of Population Health, University of Queensland and a general practitioner. He is co-editor of the *Journal of Evidence-Based Medicine*, and Chair of the Cochrane Collaboration's Methods Group on Applicability and Recommendations. As well as developing new meta-analytic methods, he has published numerous systematic reviews, including *Cochrane Reviews* in otitis media, sore throat, tonsillectomy and colorectal cancer screening.

Les Irwig is Professor of Epidemiology at the Department of Public Health and Community Medicine at the University of Sydney. His major interest is in epidemiological methods relevant to decision making. In addition to several published papers on how to review the accuracy of diagnostic tests systematically, Les Irwig was the founding chair of the Cochrane Collaboration Methods Working Group on screening and diagnostic tests and main author of its guidelines on systematic review in this area.

Chris Bain is reader in Epidemiology at the School of Population Health, University of Queensland. His research has mostly addressed the aetiology and prognosis of cancer, nutrition and disease, and health services research, with a strong emphasis on the practice and theory of systematic and quantitative reviews of health data. His own systematic reviews have covered oestrogen replacement therapy and cardiovascular disease, obesity and breast cancer, and he has contributed to a seminal international collaborative re-analysis of data on breast cancer and oral contraceptive use.

Graham Colditz is Professor in Epidemiology at the Harvard School of Public Health and Principal Investigator of the ongoing Nurses' Health Study, which follows 121 700 US women with questionnaire assessment of lifestyle factors and the use of biomarkers to assess risk of chronic diseases among women. He teaches cancer prevention, principles of screening, research synthesis/meta-analysis applications in health policy, and a course on implementing prevention.

Systematic Reviews in Health Care

A Practical Guide

Paul Glasziou
School of Population Health,
University of Queensland, Australia

Les Irwig
Department of Public Health and Community Medicine,
University of Sydney, Australia

Chris Bain
Department of Social and Preventive Medicine,
University of Queensland, Australia

Graham Colditz
Channing Laboratory, Harvard School of Public Health,
Boston, MA, USA

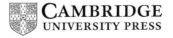

CAMBRIDGE
UNIVERSITY PRESS

PUBLISHED BY THE PRESS SYNDICATE OF THE UNIVERSITY OF CAMBRIDGE
The Pitt Building, Trumpington Street, Cambridge, United Kingdom

CAMBRIDGE UNIVERSITY PRESS
The Edinburgh Building, Cambridge CB2 2RU, UK
40 West 20th Street, New York NY 10011–4211, USA
10 Stamford Road, Oakleigh, VIC 3166, Australia
Ruiz de Alarcón 13, 28014 Madrid, Spain
Dock House, The Waterfront, Cape Town 8001, South Africa

http://www.cambridge.org

© Paul Glasziou, Les Irwig, Chris Bain & Graham Colditz 2001

First published 2001

Printed in the United Kingdom at the University Press, Cambridge

Typeface Minion 11/14.5pt   *System* Poltype® [v N]

A catalogue record for this book is available from the British Library

Library of Congress Cataloguing in Publication data
Systematic reviews in healthcare; a practical guide / Paul Glasziou . . . [et al.].
       p.   cm.
Includes bibliographical references and index.
ISBN 0 521 79962 7
1. Systematic reviews (medical research).   2. Evidence-based medicine.
3. Meta-analysis.   I. Glasziou, Paul, 1954–
R853.S94 S945   2001
610'.7'2–dc21   00-065170

ISBN 0 521 79962 7 paperback

Contents

Appendixes

Acknowledgements

This book draws substantially on material originally published as an Australian National Health and Medical Research Council (NHMRC) guide on *How to Review the Evidence: systematic identification and review of the scientific literature*. The authors wish to thank the NHMRC for their support of the work herein. We would also like to thank Sharon Saunders for assistance, Maureen Hendry, Chris Silagy, Paul O'Brien, and John McCallum for comments, and Dianne O'Connell for many of the definitions in the Glossary. We would particularly like to thank Janet Salisbury, technical writer and editor of the NHMRC edition, who was most helpful and constructive.

Introduction

Systematic literature reviews

Methods for reviewing and evaluating the scientific literature range from highly formal, quantitative information syntheses to subjective summaries of observational data. The purpose of a systematic literature review is to evaluate and interpret all available research evidence relevant to a particular question. In this approach a concerted attempt is made to identify all relevant primary research, a standardized appraisal of study quality is made and the studies of acceptable quality are systematically (and sometimes quantitatively) synthesized. This differs from a traditional review in which previous work is described but not systematically identified, assessed for quality and synthesized.

Advantages

There are two major advantages of systematic reviews (or meta-analyses). Firstly, by combining data they improve the ability to study the consistency of results (that is, they give increased power). This is because many individual studies are too small to detect modest but important effects (that is, they have insufficient power). Combining all the studies that have attempted to answer the same question considerably improves the statistical power.

Secondly, similar effects across a wide variety of settings and designs provide evidence of robustness and transferability of the results to other settings. If the studies are inconsistent between settings, then the sources of variation can be examined.

Thus, while some people see the mixing of 'apples and oranges' as a

1

problem of systematic reviews, it can be a distinct advantage because of its ability to enhance the generalizability and transferability of data.

Disadvantages

Without due care, however, the improved power can also be a disadvantage. It allows the detection of small biases as well as small effects. All studies have flaws, ranging from small to fatal, and it is essential to assess individual studies for such flaws. The added power of a systematic review can allow even small biases to result in an apparent effect. For example, Schulz et al. (1995) showed that unblinded studies gave, on average, a 17% greater risk reduction than blinded studies.

Method

A systematic review generally requires considerably more effort than a traditional review. The process is similar to primary scientific research and involves the careful and systematic collection, measurement and synthesis of data (the 'data' in this instance being research papers). The term 'systematic review' is used to indicate this careful review process and is preferred to 'meta-analysis' which is usually used synonymously but which has a more specific meaning relating to the combining and quantitative summarizing of results from a number of studies.

It may be appropriate to provide a quantitative synthesis of the data but this is neither necessary nor sufficient to make a review 'systematic'.

A systematic review involves a number of discrete steps:
- question formulation;
- finding studies;
- appraisal and selection of studies;
- summary and synthesis of relevant studies; and
- determining the applicability of results.

Before starting the review, it is advisable to develop a protocol outlining the question to be answered and the proposed methods. This is required for all systematic reviews carried out by Cochrane reviewers (Mulrow and Oxman, 1997).

Question formulation

Getting the question right is not easy. It is important to recognize that devising the most relevant and answerable question may take considerable time. Repeatedly asking 'why is this important to answer?' is helpful in framing the question correctly.

For example, are you really interested in the accuracy of the new test *per se?* Or would it be better to know whether or not the new test is more accurate than the current standard? If so, are you clear about what the current standard is?

Question formulation also involves deciding what type of question you are asking. Is it a question about an intervention, diagnostic accuracy, aetiology, prediction or prognosis, or an economic question? The multiple perspectives of health service providers, consumers and methodologists may be helpful in getting the question right.

Finding studies

The aim of a systematic review is to answer a question based on all the best available evidence – published and unpublished. Being comprehensive and systematic is important in this critical, and perhaps most difficult phase of a systematic review. Finding some studies is usually easy – finding all relevant studies is almost impossible. However, there are a number of methods and resources that can make the process easier and more productive.

Appraisal and selection of studies

The relevant studies identified usually vary greatly in quality. A critical appraisal of each of the identified potentially relevant studies is therefore needed, so that those that are of appropriate quality can be selected. To avoid a selection that is biased by preconceived ideas, it is important to use a systematic and standardized approach to the appraisal of studies.

Summary and synthesis of relevant studies

Although a quantitative synthesis is often desirable, a comprehensive and clear summary of the high-quality relevant studies to a particular question may be sufficient for synthesis and decision making. The initial focus should be on describing the study's design, conduct and results in a clear and simple manner – usually in a summary table. Following this, some summary plots are helpful, particularly if there are a large number of studies. Finally, it may be appropriate to provide a quantitative synthesis. However, as indicated above, this is neither a sufficient nor necessary part of a systematic review.

Determining the applicability of results

Following the summary and synthesis of the studies, the next step is to ask about the overall validity, strength and applicability of any results and conclusions. How and to whom are the results of the synthesis applicable? How will the effects vary in different populations and individuals?

How much work is a systematic review?

An analysis of 37 meta-analyses done by Allen and Olkin (1999) of MetaWorks, a company based in Massachusetts (USA) that specializes in doing systematic reviews, showed that the average hours for a review were 1139 (median 1110) – or about 30 person-weeks of full-time work – but this ranged from 216 to 2518 hours. The breakdown was:

- 588 hours for protocol development, searching and retrieval;
- 144 hours for statistical analysis;
- 206 hours for report writing; and
- 201 hours for administration.

However, the total time depended on the number of citations. A systematic review has a fixed component, even if there were no citations, and a variable component, which increases with the number of citations. A regression analysis of the MetaWorks analyses gives a prediction of the number of hours of work as:

$721 + 0.243x - 0.0000123x^2$ hours

where: $x =$ number of potential citations before exclusion criteria were applied.

About this book

The remainder of this book is divided into two parts:
- Part 1 includes general information on methods relevant to all systematic reviews irrespective of the type of question.
- Part 2 includes issues specific to five different question types:
  - frequency or rate of a condition or disease;
  - effects of an intervention;
  - diagnostic accuracy;
  - aetiology and risk factors; and
  - prediction and prognosis.

Appendixes A and B include details of search procedures and a listing of available software.

Part 1

General methods

The question

1.1 What types of questions can be asked?

Clinical problems and health policies may involve many different questions which need to be informed by the best available evidence. It is useful to have a classification of the different types of health care questions that we may ask:

- Phenomena: 'What phenomena have been observed in a particular clinical problem, e.g. what problems do patients complain of after a particular procedure?'
- Frequency or rate of a condition or disease: 'How common is a particular condition or disease in a specified group?'
- Diagnostic accuracy: 'How accurate is a sign, symptom or diagnostic test in predicting the true diagnostic category of a patient?'
- Aetiology and risk factors: 'Are there known factors that increase the risk of the disease?'
- Prediction and prognosis: 'Can the risk for a patient be predicted?'
- Interventions: 'What are the effects of an intervention?'

Answering each type of question requires different study designs, and consequently different methods of systematic review. A thorough understanding of the appropriate study types for each question is therefore vital and will greatly assist the processes of finding, appraising and synthesizing studies from the literature. A summary of the appropriate study types for each question and of the issues that are important in the appraisal of the studies is also given in Table 1.1. General information on how to find and review studies is given in the remainder of Part 1 with further details for each question type in Part 2.

Table 1.1. *Types of clinical and public health questions, ideal study types and major appraisal issues*

Question	Ideal study types	Major appraisal issues
1. Intervention	Randomized controlled trial	Randomization Follow-up complete Blinding of patients and clinicians
2. Frequency/rate (burden of illness)	Cross-sectional study or consecutive sample	Sample frame Case ascertainment Adequate response/follow-up achieved
3. Aetiology and risk	Cohort study	Groups only differ in exposure Outcomes measurement Reasonable evidence for causation
4. Prediction and prognosis	Cohort study	Inception cohort Sufficient follow-up
5. Diagnostic accuracy	Random or consecutive sample	Independent, blind comparison with 'gold standard' Appropriate selection of patients
6. Phenomena	Qualitative research	Appropriate subject selection and methods of observation

1.1.1 Interventions

An intervention will generally be a therapeutic procedure such as treatment with a pharmaceutical agent, surgery, a dietary supplement, a dietary change or psychotherapy. Some other interventions are less obvious, such as early detection (screening), patient educational materials or legislation. The key characteristic is that a person or his or her environment is manipulated in order to benefit that person.

To study the effects of interventions, it is necessary to compare a group of patients who have received the intervention (study group) with a comparable group who have not received the intervention (control group). A randomized controlled trial (RCT), which is a trial in which subjects are randomly allocated to the study or control groups, is usually the ideal design. A hierarchy of designs for the study of the effects of interventions is illustrated in Table 1.2.

1.1.2 Frequency or rate

How common is a particular feature or disease in a specified group in the population? This is measured as the frequency (proportion or prevalence) or rate (incidence) of the feature or disease. For example, the prevalence of osteoarthritis with ageing, or the rate of new cases of human immunodeficiency virus (HIV).

The appropriate study design in this case is a cross-sectional survey with a standardized measurement in a representative (e.g. random) sample of people; for a rate, the sample would need to be followed over time. If, instead of a single frequency, we become interested in the causes of variation of that frequency, then this becomes a question of risk factors or prediction (see below).

1.1.3 Diagnostic accuracy

How accurate is a particular diagnostic screening test? If there is good randomized trial evidence that an intervention for a particular condition works then it may be necessary to assess how accurately the condition can be diagnosed from a sign, symptom or diagnostic test. To do this, a comparison is needed between the test of interest and a 'gold standard' or reference standard. The most commonly used measures of accuracy are the sensitivity and specificity of the test.

If we move from an interest in accuracy to an interest in the effects on patient outcomes, then the question becomes one of intervention (that is, the effects on patients of using or not using the test, as is the case for population screening). However, we are generally content to use diagnostic accuracy as a surrogate to predict the benefits to patients.

Table 1.2. *Types of studies used for assessing clinical and public health interventions (question 1 in Table 1.1)*

Study design	Protocol
Systematic review	Systematic location, appraisal and synthesis of evidence from scientific studies (usually randomized controlled trials)
Experimental studies	
Randomized controlled trial	Subjects are randomly allocated to groups either for the intervention/treatment being studied or control/placebo (using a random mechanism, such as coin toss, random number table, or computer-generated random numbers) and the outcomes are compared
Pseudorandomized controlled trial	Subjects are allocated to groups for intervention/treatment or control/placebo using a nonrandom method (such as alternate allocation, allocation by days of the week or odd–even study numbers) and the outcomes are compared
Comparative (nonrandomized and observational) studies	
Concurrent control	Outcomes are compared for a group receiving the treatment/intervention being studied, concurrently with control subjects receiving the comparison treatment/intervention (e.g. usual or no care)
Historical control	Outcomes for a prospectively collected group of subjects exposed to the new treatment/intervention are compared with either a previously published series or previously treated subjects at the same institutions
Cohort	Outcomes are compared for groups of subjects who have been exposed, or not exposed, to the treatment/intervention or other factor being studied
Case-control	Subjects with the outcome or disease and an appropriate group of controls without the outcome or disease are selected and information is obtained about the previous exposure to the treatment/intervention or other factor being studied
Interrupted time series	Trends in the outcome or disease are compared over multiple time points before and after the introduction of the treatment/intervention or other factor being studied

Table 1.2. (*cont.*)

Study design	Protocol
Other observational studies	
Case series	A single group of subjects are exposed to the treatment/intervention
Post-test	Only outcomes after the intervention are recorded in the case series, so no comparisons can be made
Pretest/post-test	Outcomes are measured in subjects before and after exposure to the treatment/intervention for comparison (also called a 'before-and-after' study)

1.1.4 Risk factor or aetiology

Is a particular factor, such as patient characteristic, laboratory measurement, family history, etc., associated with the occurrence of disease or adverse outcomes? To answer this question a clear association between the factor and the disease must first be established. The most appropriate study type is a long-term follow-up of a representative inception cohort.

If a clear association is shown, the next stage is to determine whether that association is causal. That is, whether the factor under consideration causes the disease or outcome of interest or is merely associated with it for other reasons. This involves issues beyond the degree of association, such as the dose–response relationship and biological plausibility.

1.1.5 Prediction and prognosis

Based on one or several risk factors, what is the level of risk for a particular outcome to the person? Unlike the question of aetiology, causation is not so crucial. Strongly predictive risk markers are also useful. The most appropriate study type is a long-term follow-up of a representative inception cohort.

1.1.6 Phenomena

This question seeks to know the phenomena, subjective and objective, associated with a particular clinical situation. This represents the beginnings of studying a situation by simple observation or questioning. A common research method in health care is qualitative research, that is, the observation and questioning of patients about their experience. We will not cover the systematic reviewing of such questions in this book.

1.2 What is the relevant question?

A well-formulated question generally has four parts:
- the population (or patient group);
- the intervention (e.g. the treatment, test or exposure);
- the comparison intervention (optional, and defaults to no treatment, no test or no exposure if no comparison given); and
- the outcomes.

This question structure is known by the acronym PICO.

Since we will often be interested in all outcomes, the first two parts of the question may be sufficient (see Section 2.2).

1.3 How focused should the question be?

The question should be sufficiently broad to allow examination of variation in the study factor (e.g. intensity or duration) and across populations. For example:

What is the mortality reduction in colorectal cancer from yearly faecal occult blood screening in 40–50-year-old females?

is too narrow as an initial question.

However:

What is the effect of cancer screening on the general population?

is clearly too broad and should be broken down into cancer-specific screening questions.

A better question may be:

What is the mortality reduction in colorectal cancer from faecal occult blood screening in adults?

as this allows the effects of screening interval, age group and gender to be studied.

2

Finding relevant studies

Finding all relevant studies that have addressed a single question is not easy. There are currently over 22 000 journals in the biomedical literature. MEDLINE indexes only 3700 of these, and even the MEDLINE journals represent a stack of over 200 metres of journals per year.

Beyond sifting through this mass of published literature, there are problems of duplicate publications and accessing the 'grey literature', such as conference proceedings, reports, theses and unpublished studies. A systematic approach to this literature is essential in order to identify all of the best evidence available that addresses the question.

As a first step, it is helpful to find out if a systematic review has already been done or is under way. If not, published original articles need to be found.

2.1 Finding existing systematic reviews

Published reviews may answer the question, or at least provide a starting point for identifying the studies. Finding such reviews takes a little effort. A general MEDLINE search strategy proposed by McKibbon et al. which is relevant to all question types is given in Appendix A. However, for interventions, a check should also be made of the Cochrane Library for a completed Cochrane review, a Cochrane protocol (for reviews under way) or a nonCochrane review in the Database of Abstracts and Reviews (DARE) on the Cochrane Library, compiled by the Centre for Reviews and Dissemination at York (United Kingdom).

2.2 Finding published primary studies

It is usually easy to find a few relevant articles by a straightforward literature search, but the process becomes progressively more difficult as we try to identify additional articles. Eventually, you may sift through hundreds of articles in order to identify one further relevant study. This is the result of a phenomenon observed when the number of journals with articles on a topic is arranged by how many articles on that topic they contain: this is known as Bradford's law of scattering. It's implication is that, as a scientific field grows, the literature becomes increasingly scattered throughout journals and more difficult to organize. This phenomenon has been demonstrated with the literature on acquired immunodeficiency syndrome (AIDS) (Self et al., 1989). In 1982, there were only 14 journals that had literature on AIDS. By 1987 this had grown to more than 1200. The authors observed the cumulative percentage of journal titles versus journal articles for AIDS and found a Bradford distribution, with the first third of articles in 15 journals, the second third in 123 journals and the final third in 1032 journals.

There are no magic formulae to make this process easy, but there are a few standard tactics which, together with the assistance of a librarian experienced with the biomedical literature, can make your efforts more rewarding.

2.2.1 Breaking down study question into components

A central tactic is to take a systematic approach to breaking down the study question into components using a Venn diagram. The Venn diagram for the question 'What is the mortality reduction in colorectal cancer from faecal occult blood screening in adults?' is shown in Figure 2.1.

Once the study question has been broken into its components, they can be combined using 'AND' and 'OR'. For example, in Figure 2.1:

- (mortality AND screen) represents the overlap between these two terms and retrieves only articles that use both terms. A PubMed search using the terms mortality AND screen retrieves 564 articles (at the time of all searches: new citations are added to the PubMed database regularly).
- (screen AND colorectal neoplasm AND mortality) represents the small area where all three circles overlap and retrieves only articles with all three terms. A PubMed search using these three terms retrieves 37 articles.

Question: What is the mortality reduction in colorectal cancer from
faecal occult blood screening in adults?

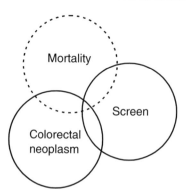

Figure 2.1   Venn diagram for colorectal screening.

- (screen AND (mortality OR survival)) retrieves articles when the
  term screening and either mortality or survival appears in the record.
  A PubMed search using the terms screen AND (mortality OR survival) retrieves 907 articles.

Complex combinations are possible. For example, the following combination captures all the overlap areas between the circles:

- (mortality AND screen) OR (mortality AND colorectal neoplasms)
  OR (screen AND colorectal neoplasms): using this combination of
  terms, a PubMed search retrieves 7928 articles.

Although the overlap of all three parts will generally have the best
concentration of relevant articles, the other areas may still contain
many relevant articles. Hence, if the disease AND study factor combination (solid circles in Figure 2.1) is manageable, it is best to work with
this and not further restrict by, for example, using outcomes (broken
circle in Figure 2.1).

2.2.2 Use of synonyms

When the general structure of the question is developed, it is worth
looking for synonyms for each component. This process is illustrated in
Table 2.1.

Table 2.1. *Using synonyms of components of the three-part question to devise a literature search*

Question: What is the mortality reduction in colorectal cancer from faecal occult blood screening in adults?

Question part	Question term	Synonyms
Population/setting	Adult, human	
Study factor	Screening, colorectal cancer	Screen*[b], early detection, bowel cancer
Outcome[a]	Mortality	Death *[b], survival
Ideal design[a]	Methodological terms	

[a] Both outcome and design are options which are only needed when the search results are unmanageable.
[b] Wildcard symbol (finds words with the same stem).

Thus, a search string might be:

(screen* OR early detection) AND (colorectal cancer OR bowel cancer) AND (mortality OR death* OR survival)

The term 'screen*' is shorthand for words beginning with screen, e.g., screen, screened, screening, etc. (Note: the wildcard symbol varies between systems, e.g. it may be an asterisk (*), or colon (:).)

Similar terms may be generated by thinking both up and down the hierarchy of abstraction, that is, by being less and more specific. For example, 'early detection' is a more general term than screening. More specific terms would be specific screening tests such as faecal occult blood, sigmoidoscopy, colonoscopy, etc.

In looking for synonyms you should consider both text words and key words in the database. The MEDLINE keyword system, known as MeSH, has a tree structure that covers a broad set of synonyms very quickly. The 'explode' (exp) feature of the tree structure allows you to capture an entire subtree of MeSH terms within a single word. Thus, for the colorectal cancer term in the above search, the appropriate MeSH term might be:

colonic neoplasm (exp)

The 'explode' incorporates all the MeSH tree below colonic neoplasm, viz.

colorectal neoplasms
  colonic polyps
    adenomatous polyposis coli
  colorectal neoplasms
    colorectal neoplasms, hereditary nonpolyposis
  sigmoid neoplasms

While the MeSH system is useful, it should supplement rather than usurp the use of textwords so that incompletely coded articles are not missed.

2.2.3 Snowballing

The process of identifying papers is an iterative one. It is best to devise a strategy on paper initially, as illustrated in Table 2.1. However, this will inevitably miss useful terms, and the process will need to be repeated and refined. The results of the initial search are used to retrieve relevant papers, which can then be used in two ways to identify missed papers:
- the bibliographies of the relevant papers can be checked for articles missed by the initial search; and
- a citation search, using the Science Citation Index (www.isinet. com/), can be conducted to identify papers that have cited the identified relevant studies, some of which may be subsequent primary research.

Studies missed by your search (but found through references or experts) provide invaluable clues for improving your search

These missed papers are invaluable – they provide clues on how the search may be broadened to capture further papers (e.g. by studying the MeSH keywords that have been used). The whole procedure may then be repeated using the new keywords identified. This iterative process is sometimes referred to as 'snowballing'.

2.2.4 Handsearching

If the relevant articles appear in a limited range of journals or conference proceedings, it may be feasible and desirable to search these by hand. This is obviously more important for unindexed or very recent journals, but may also pick up relevant studies not easily identified from title or abstracts. Fortunately, the Cochrane Collaboration is systematically handsearching a number of journals to identify controlled trials and a master list is maintained on the Internet (www.cochrane.org/). This should be checked before undertaking your own handsearch. However, for other question and study types there has been no such systematic search.

2.2.5 Methodological terms

MEDLINE terms not only cover specific content but also a number of useful terms on study methodology. For example, if we are considering questions of therapy, many randomized trials are tagged in MEDLINE by the specific methodological term:

> randomized-controlled-trials in [publication type]

or as:

> controlled-clinical trials in [publication type]

(Note that use of 'ize' spelling of randomized is necessary when using MEDLINE.) However, many studies do not have the appropriate methodological tag. The Cochrane Collaboration and the United States National Library of Medicine (NLM) are working on correctly retagging the controlled trials, but this is not the case for other study types.

2.2.6 Methodological filters

An appropriate methodological filter may help confine the retrieved studies to primary research. For example, if you are interested in whether screening reduces mortality from colorectal cancer (an intervention), then you may wish to confine the retrieved studies to controlled trials. The idea of methodological terms may be extended to multiple terms that attempt to identify particular study types. One very useful tool for a noncomprehensive but good initial search is available using the NLM's free Internet version of MEDLINE PubMed – the Clinical Queries section (www.ncbi.nlm.nih.gov/PubMed/clinical.html) which has inbuilt search filters based on methodological search techniques developed by Haynes et al. (1994). The filters are described in Appendix A. They offer four study categories (aetiology, prognosis, treatment, diagnosis) and the choice of emphasizing sensitivity or

> Efficient search =
> content terms +
> methodological
> filter

specificity in the search. Other methodological filters are discussed in Part 2 for each type of question.

2.2.7 Use of different databases

There are a number of other databases apart from MEDLINE; selection depends on the content area and the type of question being asked. For example, there are databases for nursing and allied health studies, such as CINHAL and for psychological studies such as Psyclit. If it is a question of intervention, then the Controlled Trials Registry within the Cochrane Library is a particularly useful resource. This issue is further discussed in the specific question types in Part 2 of this book.

One database is never enough

2.2.8 What about multiple languages?

Studies are conducted in all parts of the world and published in different languages. So should a systematic review seek to find all materials published in all languages? The systematic reviewer has two options. Firstly, to try to identify all relevant studies irrespective of the country in which they were conducted or the language in which they have been published. This option, however, is generally difficult with current electronic databases. An alternative is to consider restricting the inclusion criteria by the country in which the studies were conducted, which will still provide an unbiased sampling frame of studies. However, to include studies only in, say, English would lead to greater bias as positive studies conducted in countries of nonEnglish-speaking backgrounds are more likely to be submitted to an English-speaking journal and hence this exaggerates the usual publication bias with a 'tower of Babel' bias. Hence, the reviewer should be cautious about including studies published in English but conducted in a nonEnglish-speaking country unless there is also an intensive search for other studies conducted in that country and not published in English.

2.2.9 Summary

Time and careful thought are invaluable in developing an efficient search strategy. The search itself may be summarized as:

Good search = PICO + FILTER

But the use of multiple strategies is important to track down all articles.

2.3 Finding unpublished primary studies

To reduce publication bias (see Section 2.4), it is important to search for unpublished studies. There are two approaches to finding unpublished studies: searching relevant databases and contacting experts.

2.3.1 Search relevant databases

An appendix in the *Cochrane Handbook* (available on the Cochrane Library CD) contains a list of about 30 clinical trials registries with completed and ongoing studies registered in specialized areas such as AIDS and cancer.

For other question types, information will be more difficult to find, but any available databases should be checked – in particular, research funding bodies may be able to provide a list of research. However, this has rarely been systematically compiled outside controlled trials. An exception is the International Agency for Research on Cancer (IARC) bibliography of ongoing cancer epidemiology research (Sankaranarayanan et al., 1996). The website www.controlled-trials.com provides a meta-register of controlled trials and online access to a comprehensive listing of ongoing and completed controlled trials in all areas of health care.

2.3.2 Writing to experts

Another option is to contact the principal investigators of relevant studies directly, asking whether they know of additional studies.

However, the usefulness of writing to experts varies. An analysis of a recent review of the value of near-patient testing (that is, diagnostic tests that can be done entirely at the clinic, such as dipstick urine tests; McManus et al., 1998) showed that, of 75 papers eventually identified, nearly one-third were uniquely identified by contacting experts. The

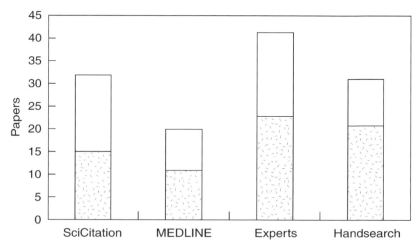

Figure 2.2   Papers identified by different search methods in a systematic review of near-patient testing. Shaded columns, unique; open columns, not unique.

data are shown in Figure 2.2, which also illustrates the general point that it is worth using multiple sources. However, near-patient testing is an area of emerging technology, and a larger proportion than usual of papers were possibly unpublished, published in less common sources or presented at conferences.

2.4 Publication bias – a crucial problem

2.4.1 What is publication bias?

If 'positive studies' are more likely to be published than 'negative' studies then any review (traditional or systematic) of the published literature must be biased towards a 'positive' result. This is the essence of publication bias – the positive correlation between the results of the study and our ability to find that study. For example, a follow-up of 737 studies approved by the Institutional Review Board at Johns Hopkins University found that the odds ratio for the likelihood of publication of positive compared with negative studies was 2.5 (Dickersin et al., 1992). Interestingly, most nonpublication was because authors failed to submit, rather than that journals rejected 'negative' studies (Stern and Simes, 1997).

Table 2.2. *Comparison of published and registered studies for multiagent versus single-agent chemotherapy for ovarian cancer*

	Published studies	Registered studies[a]
Number of studies	16	13
Survival ratio	1.16	1.05
95% confidence interval	1.06–1.27	0.98–1.12
Probability (*P*-value)	0.02	0.25

[a] Studies registered in a clinical trial registry at initiation (i.e. before the results were known).
Data from Simes (1987).

2.4.2 Does this affect the results of the reviews?

Systematic exclusion of unpublished trials from a systematic review introduces bias if the unpublished studies differ from the published, e.g. because of the statistical significance or the direction of results. In a review of multiagent versus single-agent chemotherapy for ovarian cancer, Simes (1987) found statistically and clinically different results for 16 published studies and 13 studies that had been registered in a clinical trials register, some of which were published and some not (Table 2.2). Since the registered trials were registered at inception rather than completion, their selection for inclusion in the review is not influenced by the outcome of the study, therefore they constitute an incomplete *but unbiased* set of studies. Several studies (Clarke and Hopewell, 2000) have demonstrated that the publication bias can also be viewed as a publication delay. That is, positive trials tend to be written up, submitted and published earlier than 'negative' trials. Hence, this problem is likely to occur earlier in the development of the technology, whereas as it matures there is a steady drift to all the studies being published and a diminution of the effects of publication bias. This is important to consider in looking at both published and registered studies, as even with registry studies the results may be biased by the delay in access to the results.

2.4.3 What can we do about publication bias?

It is vital that eventually all clinical trials are registered at their inception so that systematic reviews and recommendations about therapy can be made on the basis of all relevant research, and not a biased subset. In the meantime we must settle for making our best efforts at retrieving the grey literature.

These methods include using existing clinical trials registries (a list of registries and their contact details are available in the *Cochrane Handbook* in the Cochrane Library), scanning major conference proceedings and contacting experts and researchers working in the area of a particular question to ask if they know of other relevant published or unpublished research. In Chapter 4, on synthesis of the studies, we will also describe some methods of identifying the potential significance of publication bias based on the identified studies, such as 'funnel' plots. However, these only help to diagnose the problem of bias, not to cure or prevent it.

2.4.4 Duplicate publications

The converse of an unpublished study is a study that is published several times. This is often, but not always, obvious. For example, in a review of the effect of the drug ondansetron on postoperative vomiting, Tramer et al. (1997) found 17% of trials had duplicate reports. Nine trials of oral ondansetron were published as 14 reports, and 19 trials of intravenous ondansetron were published as 25 reports. One multicentre trial had published four separate reports with different first authors. Most surprisingly, four pairs of identical trials had been published that had nonoverlapping authorships!

Unfortunately, there is no simple routine means of detecting such duplicates except by some careful detective work. Occasionally, it will be necessary to write to the authors. Clearly, if duplicate publications represent several updates of the data, then the most recent should be used.

Publication bias means that study availability is influenced by study outcome

3

Appraising and selecting studies

Readers will naturally wish to know how good the reviewed research is and why you have excluded some studies that address the question at issue. In both situations you need to explain your judgments, which will usually be based on your assessment of study quality and applicability.

The process will usually need to be done in two stages; firstly, an initial screen for basic eligibility criteria and secondly, a detailed appraisal of quality. The eligibility screen might ask whether the study addresses the question and achieves some minimal quality criteria. For example, for an intervention question this might be evidence of a control group. This process is outlined in Figure 3.1.

3.1 Standardizing the appraisal

Providing an explicit and standardized appraisal of the studies that have been identified is important for two reasons. Firstly, a systematic review should try to base its conclusions on the highest-quality evidence available. To do this requires a valid and standardized procedure to select from the large pool of studies identified so that only the relevant and acceptable quality studies are included in the review. Secondly, it is important to convey to the reader the quality of the studies included as this indicates the strength of evidence for any recommendation made.

3.1.1 What study features should be assessed?

Overall, the study features that are most important to assess are those that involve selection and measurement bias, confounding and follow-

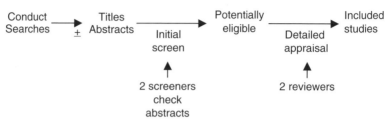

Figure 3.1   The process of appraising and selecting studies.

up of participants. In Part 2 these features are examined for each question type under the following headings:

1. Has selection bias (including allocation bias in randomized controlled trials (RCTs)) been minimized?
2. Have adequate adjustments been made for residual confounding?
3. Have the final outcomes been adequately ascertained?
4. Has measurement or misclassification bias been minimized?

3.1.2 Is it important to have a structured appraisal?

If unstructured appraisals are made, there is a tendency to look more critically at the studies whose conclusions we dislike. For example, 28 reviewers were asked to assess a single (fabricated) study but were randomly allocated to receive either the positive or negative version (Mahoney, 1977). The identical methods section of these fabricated versions was rated significantly worse by the reviewers of the negative study compared with the positive study. Hence, it is essential to appraise all papers equally. This can be done in part by using a standardized checklist. Part 2 of this book outlines the important appraisal issues for the different question types outlined in Section 1.1 and shows specific checklists for some of the question types.

These standardized checklists allow assessment of how important measurement and selection biases were avoided.

3.1.3 How many reviewers are required?

Using more than one reviewer is rather like getting a second opinion on a medical diagnosis. Because of the importance of appropriately selecting studies, at least two reviewers should be used. Each reviewer should independently read and score each of the studies that can potentially be included in the review. They should then meet to resolve any discrepancies between the scoring of the paper by open discussion about their justification for each of the scores. This discussion is a useful educational procedure in itself, which probably increases the consistency and accuracy of the appraisals of the paper.

3.1.4 Is it necessary to do the appraisal blind to the outcome of the study?

Some meta-analysts, including the late Tom Chalmers, have suggested that all appraisals should be done blind to the results of the individual study. This requires removing identification of the authors, journal and all reference to any results from the paper. Generally, the methods and the results section of the paper are sufficient to provide the information necessary for the appraisal (with the explicit outcomes 'blackened out' in the results section).

| Blind quality assessment is not proven to be worth the effort, but might be worthwhile for controversial reviews |

However, this approach is very time-consuming. The effect has been examined in two empirical studies, which suggest that the benefit, if any, in bias reduction by using the blinding process is small (Berlin, 1997). At present there is not a consensus about whether the gain is worth the effort. However, for particularly controversial and important issues, such a blinded appraisal should be considered.

3.2 Using the quality appraisal

The first and most important use of the quality appraisal will be to decide whether the study is included at all in the main analysis. For example, with a question of treatment, only RCTs may be selected. Deciding whether a study is randomized or not can be difficult, and hence it is very valuable to have reviewers to look carefully at the paper and come to a conclusion about this. Though a simple and obvious step, even minimal quality appraisal of the studies is omitted in many systematic reviews. For example, in an overview of reviews by Juni et al. (1999) only 40% of systematic reviews appeared to use any form of quality assessment.

After the decision to include or exclude the study has been made, there are three further uses for the appraisal scores or quality weights, as follows.

1. Threshold (recommended)

   If a study does not meet some prespecified quality standards then it would be excluded from the systematic review. For example, in the study of the effects of specific medication we might have specified that only randomized placebo controlled trials with more than 80% follow-up are to be included in the final analysis. Hence an appraisal of each of the studies to determine these three factors (randomization, placebo control, degree of follow-up) needs to be done. Clearly this will differ depending on the feasibility and type of question in the systematic review; for example, a placebo control or blinding may be impossible in an area of surgery and hence our criteria may be confined to randomization and adequate follow-up. Similarly, the criteria for a study of prognosis might include only the quality of the inception sample and the per cent of follow-up.

2. Grouping or sorting by design and/or quality (recommended)

   It is useful to consider an exploratory analysis on the design or quality features of studies. Studies can be categorized by design (e.g. randomized, cohort, case-control) or by important quality features (e.g. blinded versus unblinded) and then plotted in subgroups, with or without providing summary estimators for each of these design or quality groups. Does this make a difference to the results seen? For example:

   - Do the blinded studies give different results to the unblinded studies?
   - Do the studies with good randomization procedures give different results to those with doubtful randomization procedures?

   A sensitivity analysis on quality has been suggested by Detsky et al. (1992): a cumulative meta-analysis is done looking at the best single study, the best two single studies combined, the best three studies combined, etc. However, recent empirical work (Juni et al., 1999) showed that different summary quality scores give highly inconsistent results. Since flaws in one feature, such as follow-up, may not give a similar size or direction of bias to another design feature, such as blinding, analysing summary scores is problematic. Hence, we suggest the main focus should be on individual quality features.

3. Meta-regression on quality items (optional)

It is possible to extend this further by looking at all the features of quality simultaneously in a so-called meta-regression. However, because there will usually be a limited number of studies, such techniques are probably not justified in most meta-analyses.

4. Weighting by quality (not recommended)

Some analysts have suggested using the quality score to weight the contribution of particular studies to the overall estimate. This is inappropriate – it neither adjusts for nor removes the bias of poor studies, but merely reduces it slightly.

Further information on the appraisal for each question type is given in Part 2. The *Journal of the American Medical Association* Users' guides series (Guyatt et al., 1993) is also a good source of further information.

Summarizing and synthesizing the studies

4.1 Presenting the results of the studies (data extraction)

4.1.1 Tabular summary

It is helpful to produce tabular and graphical summaries of the results of each of the individual studies. An example of a summary table for an intervention question is shown in Part 2 of this book (Chapter 6, Table 6.1).

4.1.2 Graphical presentation

The most common and useful graphical presentation of the results of individual studies is a point estimate plot with the 95% confidence interval (CI) for each study (known as a 'forest plot'). A value of less than 1.0 indicates that the intervention studied is beneficial. A forest plot can be done for the relative risk reduction or a specific measure such as reduction in blood pressure. Studies should be sorted from those with the broadest to those with the narrowest confidence interval. If there is a summary estimator, this should be nearest the studies with the narrowest confidence intervals.

In addition, because studies with broad confidence intervals draw greater visual attention, it is useful to indicate the contribution of the study visually by the size of the symbol at the summary estimate. The area of the symbol should be made proportional to the precision of the study (more specifically, to the inverse of the variance of the study's estimator). This means that the diameter of each symbol is propor-

> One picture is worth a thousand confidence intervals, if the layout is properly informative

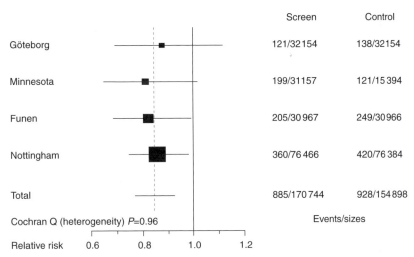

Figure 4.1   Relative mortality from colorectal cancer in screened versus unscreened (control) groups from four randomized trials of faecal occult blood screening. Dotted vertical line, the combined estimate; total, 95% confidence interval of the combined estimate. Modified from Towler et al. (1998).

tional to the inverse of the standard error of the study's estimate. These principles are illustrated in Figure 4.1, which shows the results of the systematic review of colorectal cancer screening (Towler et al., 1998).

4.2 Synthesis of study results

Except in rare circumstances, it is not advisable to pool the results of the individual studies as if they were one common large study. This can lead to significant biases because of confounding by the distribution of the study factor and the outcome factor.

However, if the studies are considered sufficiently homogenous in terms of the question and methods, and this is supported by a lack of evidence of statistical heterogeneity (see Section 4.3), then it may be appropriate to combine the results to provide a summary estimate. The method for combining studies will vary depending upon the type of questions asked and the outcome measures used. Outcome measures are summarized in Table 4.1. A further measure, the summary

Table 4.1. *Some possible outcome measures of study effects*

Outcome measures	Description
Continuous outcomes	
Difference between group means	Difference between treatment and control groups in mean values of outcome variable
Standardized difference	Differences between the treatment and control group means for each study, standardized by an estimate of the standard deviation of the measurements in that study. This removes the effect of the scale of measurement, but can be difficult to interpret
Weighted difference in means	Average (pooled) difference between treatment and control groups in mean values across a group of studies using the same scale of measurement for the outcome (e.g. blood pressure measured in mmHg)
Standardized weighted mean difference	Average (pooled) standardized difference between treatment and control groups across a group of studies, where the outcome was measured using different scales with no natural conversion to a common measure (e.g. different depression scales or different quality-of-life instruments)
Binary outcomes	
Risk difference (RD)	Difference (absolute) between treatment and control group in the proportions with the outcome. If the outcome represents an adverse event (such as death) and the risk difference is negative (below zero), this suggests that the treatment reduces the risk. In this situation the risk difference, without the negative sign, is called the absolute risk reduction
Relative risk or risk ratio (RR)	Ratio of the proportions in the treatment and control groups with the outcome. This expresses the risk of the outcome in the treatment group relative to that in the control group. If the relative risk is below 1, an adverse outcome, this suggests that the treatment reduces the risk and its complement ($1 -$ relative risk) or relative risk reduction is often used
Odds ratio (OR)	Ratio of the odds of the outcome in the treatment group to the corresponding odds in the control group. Again, for an adverse outcome, an odds ratio below 1 indicates that the treatment reduces the risk

Table 4.1. (*cont.*)

Outcome measures	Description
Hazard ratio (HR)	Ratio of the hazards in the treatment and control groups (when time to the outcome of interest is known); where the hazard is the probability of having the outcome at time t, given that the outcome has not occurred up to time t. Sometimes, the hazard ratio is referred to as the relative risk. For an adverse outcome, a hazard ratio less than unity indicates that the treatment reduces the risk
Number needed to treat (NNT)	Number of patients who have to be treated to prevent one event. It is calculated as the inverse of the risk difference without the negative sign (NNT = 1/RD). When the treatment increases the risk of the harmful outcome, then the inverse of the risk difference is called the number needed to harm (NNH = 1/RD)

Note: Further discussion of outcome measures is given in the handbook *How to Use the Evidence: Assessment and Application of Scientific Evidence* in this series (NHMRC, 1999b).

receiver-operator curve (ROC) is a measure of diagnostic test accuracy and is described in Chapter 8.

An estimate of the effect for each individual study should be obtained, along with a measure of random error (variance or standard error). The individual studies can then be combined by taking a weighted average of the estimates for each study, with the weighting being based on the inverse of the variance of each study's estimator. For example, Figure 4.1 shows, for colorectal cancer screening, the combined estimate (the dotted vertical line) and its 95% CI (the horizontal line marked 'total').

Although this principle is straightforward, a number of statistical issues make it more complicated. For example, the measures of effect have to be on a scale that provides an approximate normal distribution to the random error (e.g. by using the log odds ratio rather than just the odds ratio). Allowance must also be made for zeros in the cells of tables cross-classifying the study factor and the outcome factor, or outliers in continuous measurements. Most of the available meta-analysis software provides such methods (see Appendix B for examples of available software). Details of the properties of the various alternative statistical methods are given in Rothman and Greenland (1998). This book addresses only the general principles.

Further details of methods of synthesis for the different question types are given in Part 2. There is no single source of information for statistical methods of synthesis. The most comprehensive book currently available is the *Handbook of Research Synthesis* (Cooper and Hedges, 1994), which is particularly strong on synthesis of studies but also covers finding and appraising studies.

4.2.1 Fixed and random effects estimates

Two major categories of summary estimates are the fixed and random effects estimates. That is, is the true value a single value or does it vary across populations and circumstances?

- A fixed effect model assumes that there is a single 'true' value, which all studies are attempts to measure but with some imprecision; the fixed effect summary is a weighted average with weights proportional only to each study's precision.
- A random effects model assumes that the 'true' value varies and attempts to incorporate this variation into the weightings and the uncertainty around the summary estimate. To do this, the model first estimates the underlying study-to-study variation (which is often designated as tau (τ)), which is then included in the weighting for each study.

Mathematically, the fixed effects weights are $1/d^2$ (where d^2 is the variance of the studies estimate); the random effects weights are $1/(d^2 + \tau^2)$. From this we can see that:

- if between-study variance is small (τ is near 0) then fixed and random effects models are similar; and
- if the between-study variance is large (τ is much greater than d) then the weights for each study become almost equal.

Fixed effect and random effects models make different assumptions about the underlying data, but neither is completely correct

So which model should be used? This is best answered indirectly: if there is minimal between-study variation, the choice doesn't matter; but if there is considerable between-study variation then an explanation should be sought.

If no cause for the variation is found, then, although both models offer information, neither model is clearly correct. The fixed effects model assumes no variation when it demonstrably exists. However, the random effects model assumes the studies are a representative (or random) sample for the population of situations to which the results will be applied – a fairly unlikely assumption. So the emphasis should not be on incorporating variation but explaining it, which is discussed further in Section 4.3.

4.3 Heterogeneity and effect modification

Several factors may cause true variations in the effects seen in a systematic review. For example, the effects of a treatment may vary across different studies because of differences in:

1. the patients or the disease group, e.g. the stage or severity of disease;
2. the intervention's timing or intensity, e.g. preoperative versus postoperative chemotherapy, and the dose–response relationships;
3. the co-interventions, that is, what other treatments the patient is on; and
4. the outcome measurement and timing, e.g. there may be a delay before an effect is seen.

Unfortunately, the differences between different studies are not limited at all to these factors. Other features, such as the quality of the design and conduct of the study, the compliance with the intervention, the accuracy of the outcome measures used, etc. may cause spurious, apparent differences in different treatment effects. In turn, these spurious differences may lead us to believe that some other factor is causing true effect modification. Hence, it is important firstly to examine and eliminate such spurious sources of differences in effect between studies before exploring the possibility of true effect modification.

> Heterogeneity offers an opportunity to find out why effects vary

4.3.1 Assessing heterogeneity

The variation between studies is often considered a weakness of a systematic review but, if approached correctly, it can be a considerable strength. If the results are consistent across many studies, despite variation in populations and methods, then we may be reassured that the results are robust and transferable. If the results are inconsistent across studies then we must be wary of generalizing the overall results – a conclusion that a single study cannot usually reach. However, any inconsistency between studies also provides an important opportunity to explore the sources of variation and reach a deeper understanding of its causes and control (Thompson, 1995).

The causes of a variation in results may be due to personal factors such as gender or genes, disease factors such as severity or stage, variation in the precise methods of the intervention or diagnostic test, differences in study design or conduct, such as duration and completeness of follow-up, or the quality of measurements.

4.3.2 Measures of heterogeneity

Generally, statistical tests of heterogeneity have low power. Some variation is inevitable, and we are really more interested in the degree and causes of variation. The best current measure of the degree of variation is the between-study variance (or τ^2), which is estimated when fitting a random effects model. This has the advantage of being in the same 'units' as the results measure, e.g. if the meta-analysis looked at weight change in kilograms, then the τ is the between-study variance in kilograms. An alternative is to test for heterogeneity using the Cochran chi-square (χ^2: Cochran Q) divided by the degrees of freedom (df; number of studies -1). Values greater than 1 are indicative of heterogeneity, as follows.

- Definite heterogeneity. If the Cochran Q is statistically significant, heterogeneity must be explored. If it cannot be explained, the significant heterogeneity must be clearly stated.
- Possible heterogeneity. If the Cochran Q is not statistically significant, but Q/df is greater than 1, it is still important to explore heterogeneity.
- No heterogeneity. If the Cochran Q is not statistically significant and Q/df is less than 1, important heterogeneity is very unlikely, though effect modifications may still be present and worth exploring.

Figure 4.2 shows the results of 12 placebo-controlled trials of the effect

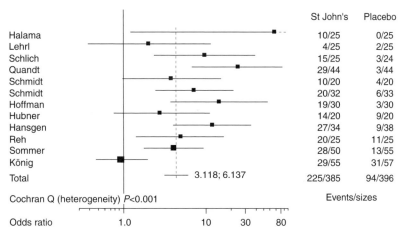

Figure 4.2   Meta-analysis of 12 placebo-controlled trials of St John's wort for depression, showing significant heterogeneity. Dotted vertical line, the combined estimate. Total, 95% confidence interval of the combined estimate. Cochran Q (odds ratio) of 34.7 on 11 degrees of freedom (df) gives $P < 0.001$.

of taking St John's wort (*Hypericum perforatum*) on depression (Linde et al., 1996). The Cochran Q is 34.7; an alternative χ^2 (Breslow and Day, 1987) is 37.9. Since there are 11 degrees of freedom (df), the Q/df ratio is 3.2 (34.7/11), indicating important heterogeneity. The *P*-value for a χ^2 of 34.7 on 11 df is < 0.001.

Even without the heterogeneity test, the graph is suspicious because the confidence interval of the largest trial (Konig) does not overlap with the confidence interval of the summary estimate.

Before exploring other sources of variation, it is important to consider whether variation may be an artefact of the outcome measure. For example, is the effect a proportional or absolute effect? If it is proportional, then measures such as the relative risk (or odds ratio or hazard ratio) or the percentage reduction (e.g. in cholesterol or blood pressure) will be appropriate. If it is absolute, then absolute risk or absolute risk reduction (risk difference) may be appropriate measures.

This question is partly biological and partly empirical. In a recent analysis of 115 meta-analyses, it was found that the absolute risk was clearly inappropriate in 30% of studies; the relative risk fared better but was still clearly inappropriate in 13% of studies (Schmid et al., 1998).

Hence, an initial check of the appropriateness of the common scale used is essential. In the St John's wort example, the Cochran Qs were 34.7 for the odds ratio, 39.0 for the relative risk and 41.6 for the risk difference. Hence, the odds ratio minimizes the Q, and appears the best choice, but clearly important heterogeneity remains.

The ideal way to study causes of true biological variation (or effect modification) is within rather than between studies, because the variation in incidental design features confounds our ability to look at true causes of effect modification (Gelber and Goldhirsch, 1987). For example, if there was one study in older men and one in younger women, then the effect of gender is confounded by the effect of age. If there was one short-term study in Caucasians and one long-term study in Chinese, then the effect of ethnicity is confounded by study duration. However, looking across studies can provide a useful initial exploratory analysis, but confirmation by combining the within-studies analysis across all studies is then desirable (see information on individual patient data meta-analysis, below).

In general, the approach to subgroup analysis and effect modification should be to assume similarity unless a difference can be demonstrated. Thus individual subgroups should *not* be tested for significance of their main effects, but should be tested for interaction to see whether the subgroups differ significantly.

The problem is illustrated in Figure 4.3, which shows a hypothetical study that is clearly statistically significant overall (the confidence interval does not cross the relative risk of 1.0). If this is now split into two subgroups (1 and 2, which each have the identical estimate), group 1 is no longer statistically significant. The correct approach here is first to test whether groups 1 and 2 are significantly different. In this case, where their point estimates are the same, it is clear that they will not differ significantly.

4.3.3 Individual patient data meta-analysis

Obtaining the original data from each study makes a number of analyses possible that are difficult or impossible if based only on summary measures from each study.

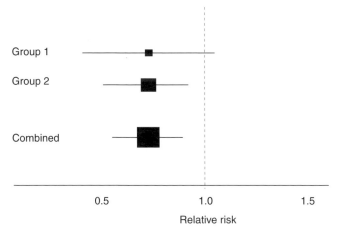

Figure 4.3   Hypothetical study showing combined and subgroup analysis: subgroups 1, 2 and the combined effect are all equivalent, but only group 2 and the combined groups are statistically significant.

For example, combined survival analysis is best done using individual patient data (Whitehead and Whitehead, 1991). As mentioned above, the ideal approach to subgroup analysis is using individual patient data. However, this usually entails much more work and collaboration, and may not be feasible. Such pooling of trial data has worked best when there is an ongoing collaboration between the triallists involved (EBCTCG, 1992).

4.4 Detecting publication bias

> Detecting publication bias is difficult; far better to avoid it

Publication bias is best avoided by improved literature searching and use of study registries (see Section 2.4). However, there are some useful diagnostic plots and statistics available that can help detect, and to some extent adjust for, publication bias.

4.4.1 Funnel plots

Smaller single-centre trials are less likely to be published, as these are more likely to be 'negative' (not statistically significant). This may be made apparent from a funnel plot that plots the size of the treatment effect against the precision of the trial (1/standard error), which is a statistical measure of the size of the study that takes into account study numbers, duration, etc. Without publication bias, this plot should be funnel-shaped – the neck of the funnel showing little spread among the larger trials, and the base of the funnel showing a wider spread among the smaller trials. With publication bias, one tail or other of the funnel may be weak or missing because the small negative trials are not present. This may be the case in Figure 4.4 of the trials of St John's wort for depression, where there is some suggestion of a publication bias. Unfortunately, this technique requires a large number of trials with a spread of sizes to provide an adequate funnel, and hence will not be helpful in many meta-analyses.

4.4.2 Statistical tests

A statistical test that is a direct analogue of the funnel plot has been developed (Begg and Mazumdar, 1994). This provides a P value for the degree of apparent bias. However, as with the graphical approach, it requires large numbers of studies – at least 25 are required for modest power. For the St John's wort example (Figure 4.4), there is a trend to bias: the P value is 0.14, but this is unreliable as it is based on only 12 studies.

4.4.3 If publication bias is suspected, what can be done?

If publication bias is suspected, the ideal method would be to estimate the degree to which bias has occurred and correct the summary estimate accordingly. Egger et al. (1997) have recently suggested a regression on an analogue of funnel plot in which the regression parameters estimate the degree of publication bias and allow a correction to be made. This is a promising line of analysis, but is unfortunately subject to a number of problems and cannot currently be recommended.

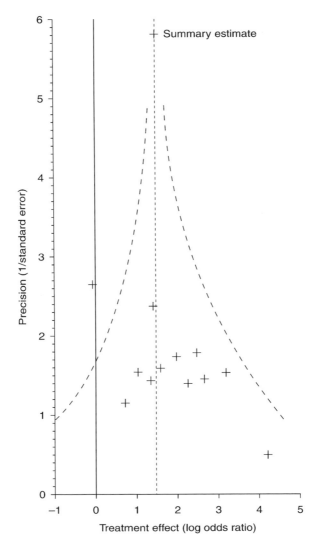

Figure 4.4   Funnel plot of 12 placebo-controlled trials of St John's wort showing some suggestion of 'missing' smaller negative trials. Dashed outer lines show boundaries of an 'ideal' funnel; if there is no heterogeneity the points are distributed evenly on either side of the summary estimate.

The file drawer number

An alternative to correcting for publication bias is a sensitivity analysis to estimate its potential impact on the conclusions. One way of doing this is to estimate the number of unpublished neutral trials of equivalent average size that would be required to make the result no longer statistically significant. This is known as Rosenthal's file drawer number (Rosenthal, 1979).

5

Applicability: returning to the question

Having completed the systematic components of the review, it is important for the reviewer to return to the original question, and assess how well it is answered by the current evidence.

- How important are study design flaws in the interpretation of the overall results?
- Is publication bias an important issue?
- If further research is needed, then specific suggestions should be made about the necessary design features rather than a simple call for more data.

To apply the results of systematic review requires more than the inclusion/exclusion criteria of the studies involved. Rather, it must be considered how a particular individual or group would differ from the study population. This clearly differs for each of the question types. Below we give a brief summary of the issues that might be considered when applying the results of intervention studies.

For questions of intervention or treatment, the issue is how the effect sizes might differ in different individuals. We suggest examining the predictors of individual response and risk, and how the risks and benefits balance varies with these. The following five-step process may be used when interpreting reviews.

1. What are the beneficial and harmful effects? Trials and meta-analysis should consider all patient-relevant endpoints potentially influenced by the treatment, including adverse effects. For example, antiarrhythmic drugs have proarrhythmic effects; anticoagulants increase the risk of bleeding. Particularly for low-risk groups, such adverse effects may be crucial. It is helpful to begin the meta-analysis by

> The inclusion/exclusion criteria are grossly insufficient to define to whom the trial results apply

45

tabulating all possible positive and negative effects of the intervention; data may or may not be available.

2. Is there predictable variation in the relative effects? Are there identifiable factors which may cause the response or effect to vary? For example,

   (a) patient features, such as age, gender, biochemical markers, etc.;
   (b) intervention factors such as the timing, compliance, or intensity of the intervention;
   (c) disease features such as hormone receptor status;
   (d) the measure of effect used: is the relative risk, risk difference, or hazard ratio most appropriate?

   Chance variation between subgroups is inevitable; hence, without prior justification and strong evidence, we should assume there is none. The evidence should come from testing whether the factor modifies the treatment effect (i.e. interaction), and *not* by testing within each individual subgroup. Ideally this is done from individual data within trials, otherwise confounding by variation in trial design may occur.

3. How do the effects vary with risk level? Low-risk patients will usually gain less absolute benefit than high-risk patients. However, we also need to know whether the relative effect, e.g. the relative risk reduction, varies with predicted event rate. If, instead of the predicted rate we use the control group event rate, there is an intrinsic negative correlation between the relative risk and the control group rate. This can be avoided by plotting the log relative risk against the log risk product (Sharp et al., 1996). If there is a change across the predicted event rate, then sophisticated statistical techniques are required to estimate the degree of change (Walter, 1997).

4. What are the predicted absolute risk reductions for individuals? The relative risk is useful for assessing the biological strength of response but, to judge whether therapy is worthwhile, we need the absolute magnitude of benefit. This might be expressed as the absolute risk reduction, or as a frequency format such as the number needed to treat (NNT): for both helping and harming). However it is expressed, it varies with the patient's expected event rate (PEER): for low-risk patients absolute benefit may not outweigh the absolute

harm. Thus, to apply the results, we also require the individual patient's expected event rate or severity based on established predictors. Information on prognosis, often external to the trial, should be used. Examples include the New Zealand guidelines on hypertension and predictors of strike risk in atrial fibrillation (Jackson, 2000).

5. Weigh up overall benefits and harms. The absolute and net benefits of therapy, and the strength of the individual patient's preferences for these, needs to be considered. If the treatment has multiple effects, e.g. adverse as well as beneficial effects, then the assessment of the absolute benefit needs to incorporate these disparate outcomes, e.g. using adjusted or threshold NNTs. If Step 4 is done well, the tradeoffs will often be clear; however, methods developed in decision analysis may be a useful supplement, e.g. quality-adjusted life years might provide summary measures when there are tradeoffs between quality and quantity of life. The central issue is whether for the individual patient the predicted absolute benefit has greater value than the harm and cost of treatment. For example, when does the reduction in strokes outweigh the risk of bleeding from anticoagulation, or when does the benefit of surgery outweigh its risk?

Even if appropriate data are lacking, it will be helpful to think through these steps qualitatively.

Questions for Part 1

1. There are several tactics to improve the quality of Internet and database searches. One seven-step approach suggests refining each search by looking specifically at:
   (a) appropriate ORs (or minuses '−');
   (b) appropriate ANDs (or pluses '+');
   (c) appropriate wildcards (such as '*');
   (d) using phrases;
   (e) avoiding problems with case-sensitivity (lower and UPPER case);
   (f) looking at links;
   (g) restricting searches to specific fields such as the title.

   An acronym for these steps is 'my plump starfish quickly lowered

Table 5.1.

Step	AltaVista	PubMed	Cochrane Library
OR	Default		
AND	+		
Wildcards	*		
Phrases	phrase		
Case			
Links			
Title	:title		

Lincoln's tie' which helps to remember the seven steps of: (a) − , (b) + , (c) *, (d) the use of quotes for phrases, (e) lower case, (f) links and (g) title. A full explanation is available at http://edweb.sdsu.edu/ WebQuest/searching/sevensteps/html.

Table 5.1 shows how the seven steps apply for the AltaVista search engine. Now complete the other two columns of the table showing how these ideas would be implemented in firstly, PubMed MED-LINE http://www.ncbi.nlm.nih.gov/entrez/query.fcgi, and secondly, the Cochrane Library.

2. The Pubmed: Clinical Queries website provides several question-specific filters: http://www.ncbi.nlm.nih.gov/entrez/query/static/ clinical.html. On the Clinical Queries home page, have a look at the link called 'this table' to see how these filters work. Now have a look at the effects on a specific search for 'indomethacin AND Alzheimer'. Compare the number of hits and the number of controlled trials you find by looking at PubMed MEDLINE www.ncbi.nlm.nih.gov/entrez/query.fcgi and PubMed Clinical Queries: www.ncbi.nlm.nih.gov/entrez/query/static/clinical.html using therapy and specific with firstly, the 'sensitive' button mark and secondly, the 'specific' button mark.

3. One way of finding unpublished or ongoing studies is to look at registries of trials. Go to the current controlled trials website (www.controlled-trials.com). You'll have to sign in but it is free. Now do a search on the meta-registry of controlled trials on Alzheimer to see whether there are any ongoing trials of antiin-flammatories (corticosteroids or nonsteroidal antiinflammatory

drugs) in Alzheimer's disease. The website also has links to other trials registries which you might like to explore.

4. Alternative spellings and misspellings can be a problem when doing literature searches. Try the following on MEDLINE and find out how many hits you get for each of the alternative spellings:

(a) hemorrhage;

(b) haemorrhage;

(c) hemorhage; and (d) haemorhage.

(Note: spellings (a) and (b) are the American and British spellings respectively whereas (c) and (d) are both misspellings.)

Part 2

Question-specific methods

This part describes additional issues and methods specific to the different types of questions: intervention, frequency, diagnostic test accuracy, risk factors and aetiology, prognosis and economic studies. Before reading the subsection of the specific question type you are interested in, we strongly recommend that you first read all of Part 1.

Some important resources for additional reading beyond these subsections are included in the appendixes.

Appendix A covers some general tips from a book by McKibbon et al. (1999), including a search method developed by Boynton et al. (1998) for finding current systematic reviews and methods for searching on specific questions.

Appendix B describes some available software for performing the calculations and plots. None of the packages available is comprehensive, and they usually focus on a single question type. Even within a single question, more than one software package may be required to provide all the calculations and plots needed.

6

Interventions

6.1 The question

There are many types of intervention that may be the subject of a systematic review, such as:

- therapy for a specific disease (e.g. aspirin to prevent stroke, surgery for coronary artery disease or cognitive therapy for depression);
- a change in a risk factor (e.g. blood pressure-lowering to prevent stroke, immunization to prevent hepatitis or publicity campaigns to reduce teenage smoking); or
- screening for earlier diagnosis (e.g. mammographic screening for breast cancer, antenatal screening for silent urinary tract infections or screening for cholesterol).

The defining feature is that some specific activity is undertaken with the aim of improving or preventing adverse health outcomes.

6.1.1 Study design

Because of their unique ability to control for confounders, known or unknown, randomized controlled trials (RCTs) generally provide the best evidence of efficacy for interventions. This section therefore focuses on systematic reviews of controlled trials; other study types for intervention will be discussed Section 9.

However, in interpreting RCTs for policy making and applying them to individuals, nontrial evidence will often be appropriate. For example, surveillance data may provide the best information on rare adverse effects, and cohort studies may provide the best information on the prognostic factors needed to predict the pretreatment risk of an individual.

6.2 Finding relevant studies

6.2.1 Finding existing systematic reviews

Appendix A gives information on finding existing systematic reviews. A check should be made of the Cochrane Database of Systematic Reviews (CDSR; Cochrane Library) and DARE databases for Cochrane and nonCochrane reviews respectively. Even if the review is not considered to be completely appropriate, its reference list will provide a useful starting point.

6.2.2 Finding published primary studies

The best search methods are changing rapidly. The efforts of the Cochrane Collaboration have been seminal in the more systematic registering, compiling and classifying of all controlled trials in databases such as MEDLINE. Use of the Cochrane Library and contact with the Collaboration would be advisable when undertaking any new review of interventions.

An initial search should use the Cochrane Controlled Trials Registry (CCTR), which is available on the Cochrane Library CD. CCTR contains a listing of potential controlled trials. These have been identified by systematically searching databases such as MEDLINE and EMBASE, by handsearching a number of journals and the specialized registers of trials that are maintained by the Collaborative Review Groups.

A registry called CENTRAL has been distributed on the CD-ROM edition of the Cochrane Library since issue 4 (1997). It contains some reports of studies that are found not to be relevant for inclusion in Cochrane reviews. It is also likely to contain duplicates and errors. It includes all records in MEDLINE that contain the publication type (pt):

> An experienced searcher will only find half the relevant trials in MEDLINE – use multiple approaches and multiple people

randomized controlled trial
OR

controlled clinical trial

CCTR is the 'clean' version of CENTRAL. Controlled trials that meet the necessary quality criteria, are assigned the keyword 'CCTR'.

Note that, whether searching CENTRAL, MEDLINE or other databases, a carefully constructed search is still required, using the structured approach described in Chapter 2, with synonyms and wildcards.

Does a search need to go beyond CENTRAL?

As the Cochrane Library is updated every 3 months, a search for more recent studies may be needed. In addition, handsearching of key journals and conference proceedings should be considered.

6.2.3 Finding unpublished studies

There are two approaches for searching unpublished studies. Firstly, an appendix in the Cochrane Handbook (available on the Cochrane Library CD) contains a list of about 30 clinical trials registries with completed and ongoing studies registered in specialized areas such as acquired immune deficiency syndrome (AIDS) and cancer. Secondly, it may be helpful to contact the principal investigators of relevant studies to ask them whether they know of additional studies.

6.3 Appraising and selecting studies

6.3.1 Standardizing the appraisal

What study features should we assess?

Numerous quality assessment methods have been used: a review in 1994 identified 25 methods (Guyatt et al., 1994). The number of items ranged from three to 34; the times for completion per study ranged between 10 and 45 minutes, and the reliability κ (which is a measure of agreement beyond that explained by chance) ranged between 0.12 and 0.95 on a scale from 0 to 1.

As the optimal use of quality items and scales is still not clear, we recommend that items be generally restricted to those that have been shown to affect the results of trials. Empirical work by Schulz et al. (1995) has shown that how well the random allocation procedure is concealed and the degree of blinding both have an important influence. These two items should be assessed in any review and are described below. A third item involving the level of patient follow-up is also important.

1. Has selection bias (including allocation bias) been minimized?

    Random allocation is crucial for creating comparable groups. However, it is the allocation concealment before randomization that is vital, rather than the randomness of the random number sequence. An assessment of the allocation concealment requires an explicit statement of method, such as a central computerized randomization system. If this is not convincing, then secondary evidence is provided by demonstrating comparability from the baseline values of the randomized groups.

2. Have adequate adjustments been made for residual confounding?

    For RCTs, the elimination of bias is closely related to avoidance of selection bias (see above) because appropriate selection/allocation minimizes bias at the sample stage. If this allocation is imperfect, however, statistical adjustments may have to be made at the post-selection stage.

3. Have the final outcomes been adequately ascertained?

    Having created comparable groups through randomization, high rates of follow-up and inclusion of all randomized patients in the analysis of outcome data ('intention-to-treat' analysis) are important. However, this control of selection bias after treatment assignment has not been empirically demonstrated to reduce bias as much as appropriate randomization and blinding. However, it is still useful to extract and report data on the degree of follow-up.

4. Has measurement or misclassification bias been minimized?

    Blinding of outcome measurements becomes more crucial as the measure becomes more subjective and hence more open to observer bias. This is particularly important for symptoms and other patient self-report measures. The use of adequate placebos generally provides adequate blinding of outcome measures, but blinding can also be achieved without placebos, e.g. by bringing in an independent 'blinded' observer to assess the outcome measure.

Appraisal checklists

Box 6.1 is an example of an appraisal checklist that includes these elements, modified from a checklist developed by Iain Chalmers (*Cochrane Handbook*; available on the Cochrane Library CD). Other appraisal methods may be used but should always include the randomization and blinding items. Other alternatives are given in Guyatt et al. (1993, 1994) and Liddle et al. (1996).

Should scales be generic or specific?

In addition to the generic items that have been discussed, some specific items may be useful in a particular analysis. For example, the precise methods used for the outcome measure are part of the quality of conduct of the study and are vital for the interpretation of the results. A trial of treatment of 'glue ear' in children, for example, may have used clinical appearance of the eardrum, tympanograms, audiograms or a combination for measures of outcome.

> Keep the appraisal items to a few simple items which have proven to be important causes of bias

6.4 Synthesis of study results

6.4.1 Presenting the results of the studies

Both the number of trials identified and selected should be reported, and the reason stated for those that are not selected. For example, reviews of treatment are often limited to properly randomized trials. Hence the number of apparent trials, and the number with proper randomization would be reported.

Summary table

The generic and specific quality items should be tabulated together with the major study characteristics, such as the nature and intensity of the intervention, the outcome measures, and the principal results, as illustrated in Table 6.1.

Box 6.1 Checklist for appraising the quality of studies of interventions

1. Method of treatment assignment
   (a) Correct, blinded randomization method described OR randomized, double-blind method stated AND group similarity documented
   (b) Blinding and randomization stated but method not described OR suspect technique (e.g. allocation by drawing from an envelope)
   (c) Randomization claimed but not described and investigator not blinded
   (d) Randomization not mentioned

2. Control of selection bias after treatment assignment
   (a) Intention to treat analysis AND full follow-up
   (b) Intention to treat analysis AND $< 15\%$ loss to follow-up
   (c) Analysis by treatment received only OR no mention of withdrawals
   (d) Analysis by treatment received
       AND no mention of withdrawals
       OR more than 15%
       withdrawals/loss-to-follow-up/post-randomization exclusions

3. Blinding
   (a) Blinding of outcome assessor
       AND patient and care giver
   (b) Blinding of outcome assessor
       OR (patient AND care-giver)
   (c) Blinding not done

4. Outcome assessment (if blinding was not possible)
   (a) All patients had standardized assessment
   (b) No standardized assessment OR not mentioned

Source: modified from I Chalmers, *Cochrane Handbook*; available on the Cochrane Library CD-ROM.

Table 6.1. *Example summary table of quality features of a set of hypothetical intervention trials*

		Trial descriptors		Quality items			
Trial	*n*	Intervention	Population and other content-specific items[a]	Randomization procedure	Blinding	Follow-up	Results (relative risk)
1	324	20 mg daily		Central computer	Double	90% at 2 years	0.7
2	121	25 mg twice daily		Envelopes	Single	80% at 5 years	0.6
3	987	10–25 mg		Not stated	None	98% at 1 year	0.55

[a] Information relevant to particular study (e.g. information on participants, methods, outcomes).

Note: A Cochrane review generally has a summary table with author/reference, methods, participants (age, gender, etc.), interventions, outcomes, notes (quality scores may also be included).

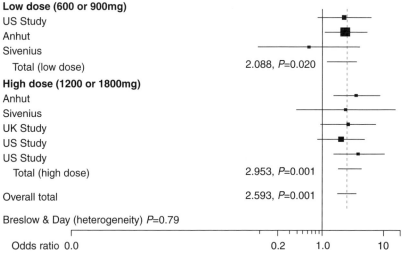

Figure 6.1		Placebo-controlled trials of treatment of epilepsy with the drug gabapentin and the relative proportions of '50% responders' (with at least 50% reduction in seizure frequency); grouped by low (600 or 900 mg) or high (1200 or 1800 mg) doses, showing a nonsignificant trend to a greater response with the higher dosage. Dotted vertical line, the combined estimate. Total, 95% confidence interval of the combined estimate.

Graphical presentation

Even if studies are not to be combined, a summary plot of the results of each is invaluable. As outlined in Section 4.1, the basic plot is a summary estimate of effect together with a confidence interval (known as a 'forest plot'). The studies may be arranged in order of date, size, quality score, strength of intervention, control event rate or several other useful attributes, but should not be arranged by the size of effect. A second attribute may be indicated by subgrouping. For example, studies might be grouped by high- or low-intensity intervention, and then by study quality within these categories. An example of a forest plot for RCTs on treatment of epilepsy with the drug gabapentin is shown in Figure 6.1.

> In summary forest plots, use 'dot' size and study order to assist the reader's interpretation

6.4.2 Synthesis of study results

For some systematic reviews, it may only be reasonable to present the table of study characteristics and basic data plots. However, if formal combination is considered appropriate, then there are two major aims to such a meta-analytic synthesis of controlled trial data. Firstly, to find a summary estimate of the overall effect, and secondly, to examine whether and how this average effect is modified by other factors.

To enable a single summary outcome measure, all the trial results must be expressed in a common metric (unit). Ideally, this should be the most patient-relevant outcome and expressed in a directly interpretable manner (e.g. reduction in the risk of death, proportional reduction in symptoms, or days of symptoms). However, the trials will not necessarily allow this, and some pragmatic choices will need to be made.

Outcome measures include discrete events (such as death, stroke or hospitalization) and continuous outcomes (such as lung function, days with headache or severity scales).

Discrete events

Discrete events can be expressed as the risk difference (RD), relative risk or risk ratio (RR), odds ratio (OR) or the average time to event (Table 4.1). The choice will depend on which measure is most stable and logical for that outcome. A useful initial guide is the L'Abbe plot

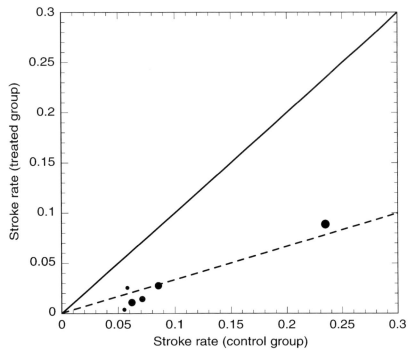

Figure 6.2   L'Abbe plot of the stroke risk in the treated group versus the stroke risk in the control group from a meta-analysis of six placebo-controlled trials of warfarin for nonvalvular atrial fibrillation. The diagonal (solid) line represents no effect. Points below this line indicate a lower rate of poor outcomes in the treated group than in the control group (i.e. benefit). The dashed line shows the overall (beneficial) effect of warfarin, which appears to increase with increasing risk in the control group.

(L'Abbe et al., 1987), which plots the event rate in the treated group against the event rate in the control group. Figure 6.2 shows the trials from a meta-analysis of six placebo-controlled trials of warfarin for nonvalvular atrial fibrillation plotted in this way.

A study of 115 meta-analyses showed that the RD varied most over different populations, whereas the RR and OR were about equally stable (Schmid et al., 1995).

An ideal approach when the time-to-event varies is survival analysis based on combined data, but the necessary data for this may not be available.

Continuous outcomes

Again, a common interpretable outcome measure is ideal. Sometimes this is impossible, in which case a common metric is needed. Examples are:

- the proportional improvement (in, say, forced expiratory volume (FEV_1) or peak flow); and

- the standardized difference – the difference between the treated and control groups divided by the standard deviation in the control group (if the treatment is likely to alter the variation; otherwise the combined estimate is more stable).

> We want to know both the average effect and variations from the average effect

6.4.3 Assessing heterogeneity

Difference in the effects seen may be caused by several factors:
- disease features, such as stage or severity;
- patient features, such as age or ethnicity;
- intensity or timing of the intervention; and, most importantly,
- study design features, such as study duration or the outcome measures used.

Even if the test for heterogeneity is nonsignificant, exploring for causes of variation is reasonable and useful. For example, in Figure 6.1 showing trials of the drug gabapentin in epilepsy, the overall test for heterogeneity was nonsignificant ($P = 0.79$), but subgrouping appeared to show a modest dose–response relationship.

6.5 Economic evaluation

Depending on the type of economic analysis required, systematic reviews of intervention studies can also provide valuable information. The basic types of economic analysis include (Drummond et al., 1997):
- cost analysis;
- cost-effectiveness analysis;
- cost–utility analyses; and
- cost–benefit analyses.

The last three all contain an effectiveness component, and hence systematic reviews will play some role. For other components, such as the cost or pricing of resources, systematic review has a limited role. Cost-effectiveness analysis is probably the most used economic analysis in Australia. For example, submissions to the Australian Pharmaceutical Benefits Scheme require a cost-effectiveness analysis (Henry, 1992; Drummond et al., 1997).

A cost-effectiveness analysis has several components, including the estimate of benefit, the change in resources utilization and the unit costs of those resources. A general formula for cost-effectiveness ratio can be written as (Drummond et al., 1997):

C–E ratio = (Costs – Savings)/Effectiveness

where: Costs = the costs of implementing the intervention; Savings = the savings from any reductions in resource use attributable to the intervention; and Effectiveness = the incremental clinical benefit gained from the intervention.

Savings result from changes in resource utilization, such as hospitalization, lengths of stay and medication usage, and are generally closely allied to clinical outcomes. Hence, systematic reviews are relevant to the estimation of the effectiveness and, usually, to the changes in resource utilization. However, the net cost (Costs – Savings) will depend on the unit costs of resources and the intervention that will vary over sites and time. Thus, direct systematic review of the C–E ratio will generally be inappropriate.

For example, for carotid endarterectomy a systematic review of the economics would first require a systematic review of the evidence of its effectiveness. This would inform us about any reductions in stroke leading to some savings. Finally, the unit costs of stroke, endarterectomy and other events would need to be established in order to calculate the net cost to be compared with the effectiveness.

6.6 Further information

This section provides only a brief overview of methods. A fuller description of the process for Cochrane systematic reviews is contained in the *Cochrane Handbook*, available as either an electronic version in the

Cochrane Library or as a hard-copy version (Mulrow and Oxman, 1996). This book is regularly updated and has become the principal source of guidance for systematic reviews of interventions.

Questions for Part 2: interventions

1. Suppose you are working at a busy suburban general practice. At lunchtime, you mention to one of your colleagues the couple of cases of children with acute otitis media you saw in the clinic that morning, and ask what the currently recommended antibiotic is. Your colleague answers that he thought that the new antibiotic guidelines suggested that antibiotics were no longer specially required. You wonder what the evidence is for this and manage to track down, through MEDLINE, a recently published systematic review in the *British Medical Journal* (Del Mar, C.B. et al. *British Medical Journal* 1997; **314**, 1526–9); this is available via the *British Medical Journal* website (www.bmj.com) at: www.bmj.com/cgi/content/full/314/7093/1526.

   (a) Before accepting the conclusions, you decide that it is worth checking that the authors did a good job of the review and, in particular, you decide to look at whether they did a thorough literature search, checked that the trials were of adequate quality and used acceptable methods for combining the studies, including looking at differences between studies and possible heterogeneity.

   (b) What methods did they use for combining the data (effect measure, fixed or random effects etc.)?

   (c) How was heterogeneity tested for? What did it show?

   (d) Were possible sources of heterogeneity explored (effect measure, design features, patient features)?

   (e) Did they explore the potential for publication bias? What methods did they use (trials registry, funnel plot, file drawer N, Begg statistic, etc.)?

   (f) What issues arise out of this meta-analysis and what further questions might the authors address?

2. Since the review in the previous question was published, a new trial

has appeared which might be added to the acute otitis media review, which examined the effects of antibiotics in younger children (Damoiseaux RA, van Balen, F.A. Hoes, A.W. Verheij, T.J. and de Melker, R.A. (2000). Primary care based randomised, double blind trial of amoxicillin versus placebo for acute otitis media in children aged under 2 years. *British Medical Journal*, **320**, 350–4). Read this article, which is available at the *British Medical Journal* website: www.bmj.com/cgi/content/full/320/7231/350.

(a) Now appraise the Damoiseaux article using the appraisal sheet given in this chapter. How does this study compare with the others already included in the review? Do you now think it is of adequate quality to be included in the meta-analysis?

(b) Obtain two of the articles in the Del Mar review (Burke, *British Medical Journal* 1991: **303**, 558–62, and van Buchem, *Lancet* 1981; 883–7) from the meta-analysis that you have examined on antibiotics as initial treatment for children with acute otitis media. Are these original studies of adequate quality? Read through both articles briefly and decide which is better. Now read the articles, using the appraisal sheet given in the chapter, to appraise conduct of the study on the four elements indicated in the sheets. Does this process alter your assessment of the studies? Do you now think they are of adequate quality to be included in the meta-analysis? What would be the ideal outcome measures for this clinical issue? Set up a data extraction form for these. Now try to extract data from the two trials.

3. Using the data in Figure 1 of the acute otitis media meta-analysis, do a combined analysis of the data (using, e.g. Meta-analyst), as follows:

(a) Set up the data in a series of 2×2 tables.

(b) Do a L'Abbe plot of the studies (plotting percentage symptom-free in the antibiotic group against the percentage symptom-free in the control group). Do you think the studies are acceptably homogeneous?

(c) Now do a formal test of heterogeneity (this is the test by the Q statistic). Are the studies homogeneous? Does this depend on the risk measure you chose?

(d) Now combine the studies and find the overall:

(i) relative risk and the relative risk reduction ($= 1 -$ relative risk);

(ii) odds ratio;

(iii) risk difference; and

(iv) number needed to treat (this can be calculated in a number of ways, e.g. directly from the $1/$ (risk difference) or from the pooled control group rate x RRR.

(e) What are the other possible sources of heterogeneity?

4. Formulate a question that you might subject to a systematic review. Is it the right question? Is it sufficiently focused as to be answerable (use the PICO format discussed in Chapter 1)? Once you have settled on an appropriate question, then write an outline of a protocol for your review. Specifically,

(a) How will you find all relevant studies? Which databases will you search? How will you find articles missed by this search?

(b) How will you appraise and select the studies? What articles will be acceptable in the review? What items will you check in each study?

(c) What endpoints will you combine in any quantitative synthesis? How will the results be combined?

Frequency and rate

7.1 The question

Questions of frequency (or prevalence) arise commonly in health care. For example:

- What is the frequency of hearing problems in infants?
- What is the prevalence of Alzheimer's disease in the over-70s?
- What is the frequency of *BrCa1* gene for breast cancer in women?

If the proportion changes over time, then a time period is incorporated into the definition to give a rate (or incidence). Thus, a possible question may be:

- What is the rate of incidence of influenza in different seasons and years?

Traditionally, for diseases, prevalence is distinguished from incidence and the following quantities have been defined (Rothman and Greenland, 1998):

- prevalence – the proportion of people who have the condition at a specific point in time (frequency of current cases);
- incidence – the instantaneous rate of development of new cases (also known as the incidence rate or simply the rate); and
- incidence proportion – the proportion of people who develop the condition within a fixed time period (also called cumulative incidence, with a specific example being the lifetime risk).

Incidence and prevalence are linked by the duration of illness, so that in a steady-state population:

Prevalence = incidence × duration

In this book, the terms 'frequency' and 'rate' are preferred to 'preva-

Prevalence,
incidence, risk and
rate are related
but different: be
clear which *you*
need to measure
and which *the
study* measured

lence' and 'incidence' because not all questions refer to diseases, but
may refer to risk factors such as diet, or false-positive rates (for diagnostic questions), and so on. The definition and calculation of frequencies
and rates involve a number of subtleties, which are described by
Rothman and Greenland (1998).

The apparent frequency may be greatly influenced by the case definition. For example, whether or not silent myocardial infarction (incidentally detected by later ECGs) is included in estimates of myocardial
infarction will change both the frequency and rate. Similarly, the precise
measurements used can be influential; for example, different rates of
deep venous thrombosis may be obtained from an ultrasound to those
obtained from a venogram. Of particular note is that, if the true
frequency is zero, the apparent frequency will consist of just the false
positives, and thus be (1 – specificity). Hence it is important for any
systematic review of frequencies to document both the population and
the definitions and measures used.

7.1.1 Study design

The aim of a study of frequency or rate is to measure a representative
sample of the target population. For frequency, this will be a random
sample survey (or census) of the target population; for rate there is an
additional requirement that the representative group be followed over
time. Thus the major study designs are (cross-sectional) surveys for
frequency, and cohort studies for rate. If the sample includes the entire
population, then these become a census (for frequency) or a disease/
condition registry (for rate).

7.2 Finding relevant studies

7.2.1 Finding existing systematic reviews

Publication is less
likely with
frequency studies,
so you may need
to look for agency
reports

There have been a few systematic reviews of frequency and rates.
However, it is still worth searching using the general methods: Appendix A gives information on finding existing systematic reviews. This
would need to be combined with content-specific terms for the disease
or risk factor being reviewed together with the terms in the next section.

7.2.2 Finding published primary studies

Unfortunately, most relevant studies are not coded as such in MED-LINE. The search requires three components:

- the alternative terms:
  incidence OR rate OR
  frequency OR proportion OR prevalence
- the condition of interest (and any synonyms), preferably using a MeSH term (exploded if possible and appropriate); and, if the number of potential studies is too large,
- a methodological filter to confine this to appropriate studies of frequency, such as random or consecutive; or the filter could focus on an appropriate 'gold standard', such as audiometry for childhood hearing problems.

Various combinations of the above three components may be used. For example, a MEDLINE search for the causes of chronic cough might use:

chronic NEAR cough

where the special search term 'NEAR' means that the 'chronic' and 'cough' need to be close together but allows for terms such as 'chronic nonproductive cough'.

This might then be restricted to references with an appropriate sample, i.e. a random or consecutive set of cases, plus an adequate gold standard test or tests, and an appropriate follow-up (to catch missed or mistaken diagnoses). Together, these give the following search:

chronic NEAR cough AND (investigat* OR diagnos* OR cause*) AND (consecutive OR follow-up OR followup)

7.2.3 Finding unpublished studies

In addition to writing to authors of published work, it is important to consider whether any government or nongovernment agencies might have relevant surveys or registries. For example, if you are interested in cancer incidence then cancer registries are an obvious source; if you are interested in communicable diseases, state or territory health departments should be contacted. Groups and societies interested in specific diseases, such as diabetes, heart disease, and cystic fibrosis, may also have done their own surveys.

7.3 Appraising and selecting studies

7.3.1 Standardizing the appraisal

What study features should we assess?

There are no standard accepted quality scales for studies of proportions. However, the principal issues are similar to those described for controlled trials of interventions (see Section 6.3).

1. Has selection bias been minimized?

   Random selection is important to obtain a representative sample. While simple random sampling is often appropriate, other methods include stratified random sampling and cluster sampling. The important issues are the definition and establishment of an appropriate sample frame and some form of random sampling.

2. Have adequate adjustments been made for residual confounding?

   The issue of confounding is not relevant to frequency and rate studies.

3. Have the final outcomes been adequately ascertained?

   Having obtained a representative group by random sampling, a high response rate is needed to maintain the representativeness and avoid bias. This is particularly important if nonresponse is associated with the condition of interest. For example, if you want to know the proportion of discharged psychiatric patients who relapsed within a year, then high follow-up is important as difficult-to-follow patients often have worse outcomes.

4. Has measurement or misclassification bias been minimized?

   As discussed in the introduction, a clear definition of the condition and the measurements used is crucial, as this will influence the apparent rate.

Table 7.1. *Example summary table of a set of hypothetical studies of frequency*

Trial	Setting	Measures	Population/ inclusion criteria	Selection	Response (%)	Results n/N (%)
1	Community	Single BP	Age 16–75	Random sample	70	10/195 (10%)
2	GP clinic	Average of 3 BP	All ages	Consecutive cases	80	30/240 (13%)
3	Skin clinic	Average of 2BP on two occasions	Age 20–65	Consecutive cases	98	4/20 (20%)

BP, blood pressure measurements.

7.4 Summarizing and synthesizing the studies

7.4.1 Presenting the results of the studies

Summary table

A systematic description of the definitions and measurements used is critical to the comparison of studies. Hence an initial summary table is crucial, like that shown in Table 7.1. The table should detail precise definitions of cases and the type and frequency of measurements used, e.g. the average of three blood pressure measurements taken in the supine position two days apart using a mercury sphygmomanometer. In addition, other potential differences between the populations should be described (e.g. gender mix, age range and other inclusion and exclusion criteria).

Graphical presentation

As with all systematic reviews, plots of the data are invaluable. For frequency and rate questions, the estimate and confidence interval should be plotted against any factors that may be predictive of the results, i.e. those elements provided in the descriptive table. For example, Figure 7.1 shows a graph of the rates of antibiotic resistance in *Propionibacterium acnes*, suggesting a trend with time, though clearly other explanations (such as measurement or populations) would need to be examined.

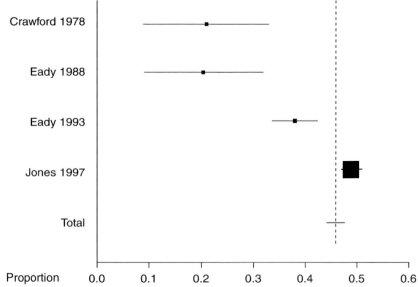

Figure 7.1   Proportion of patients with antibiotic resistance in *Propionibacterium acnes* for four studies, listed by publication date. Data from Cooper (1998).

7.4.2 Synthesis of study results

Among a group of acceptably similar studies, the methods of quantitative synthesis are relatively straightforward. If the frequencies are considered to arise from a single common population (a fixed effect model), then simple pooling will be sufficient. For example, if the prevalence of a disease was similar in all states, then an estimate of the national average prevalence would simply pool all the state disease cases, and the national prevalence (frequency) would be the total cases in the total population. The results should be reported as an overall frequency or rate and confidence interval.

However, if there is variation by case definition, measurements, population or other factors, then more complex methods are required. The first step is to look for causes of variation that may be artefacts, such as different measurements, and if possible to correct or adjust each estimate. If there appear to be true differences in the studies and populations then this should be reported. If an overall estimate is still needed, then the method depends on the aim, but may require a random effects model.

7.4.3 Assessing heterogeneity

A test for heterogeneity should be performed. Whether or not the result is significant, it is worthwhile checking whether subgroups of studies differed because of measurement method or sample frame.

Questions for Part 2: frequency

1. Should we screen for intracranial aneurysms (a ballooning of an artery in the brain)? You are on a panel discussing this question, and one important question to answer is the frequency of intracranial aneurysms. A search of the literature uncovers an article that reviews 23 studies: Rinkel, G.J.E., Djibuti, M., Algra, A. and van Gijn, J. (1998). Prevalence and risk of rupture of intracranial aneurysms: a systematic review. *Stroke*, **29**, 251–6. This article is also available on the Internet at: http://stroke.ahajournals.org/content/vol29/issue1/.
   (a) What are the strengths and weaknesses of this paper?
   (b) Do you think they have done an adequate search? an adequate appraisal? an adequate synthesis?
2. In the Rinkel paper, Figure 1 gives a summary of the prevalence including four subgroups based on the study methods (autopsy versus angiography; retrospective versus prospective). Why do you think the methods give different results? Which do you consider to be the most accurate result?
3. Using the data in the Rinkel paper, derive the summary prevalence in two different ways: firstly, pooling the results, that is, simply adding together the numbers of aneurysms and numbers of subjects; and secondly, taking a prevalence figure from each study separately and then using equal weights to combine the studies. How different are the answers? Which answer do you think is better, and why?

8

Diagnostic tests

8.1 The question

Although the principles are similar across all types of study question, systematic review of diagnostic tests requires some different approaches, notably in the methods used for combining data from different studies. As with the other types of questions, the starting point for diagnostic studies is an appropriate question, including a description of:

- the disease of interest;
- the test(s) of interest;
- patient features that are likely to alter the test performance characteristics; and
- the performance characteristics of the test compared to the performance characteristics of another test or tests.

If test performance characteristics vary between patient subgroups, this needs to be taken into account when applying the results of a systematic review of diagnostic tests. Common features that affect test performance characteristics include the symptoms, signs, tests and previous triage through the health care system that has got patients to the point at which you wish to evaluate the performance characteristics of a test. This issue is explored further in Section 8.3 on appraising the quality and applicability of studies.

Diagnostic test studies usually measure accuracy (test performance) rather than outcomes (management performance)

When the performance characteristics of the test are compared to the performance characteristics of another test(s), the situation is analogous to trials in which an intervention is compared to a placebo or to another drug. For example, we may not want to know if the presence of leukocytes in an abdominal fluid aspiration has a high sensitivity and

74

specificity for the diagnosis of appendicitis in people presenting with abdominal pain. Rather, we may want to know its incremental sensitivity and specificity compared to other features that are more easily obtained, for example, rebound tenderness in the right iliac fossa (Caldwell and Watson, 1994).

8.1.1 Study design

The ideal design for studies of diagnostic test performance is usually a cross-sectional study in which the results of tests on consecutively attending patients are cross-classified against disease status determined by a reference (gold) standard. If this is not feasible, patients should be randomized to different tests. Occasionally, the sample will be followed over time if the test is predictive of a reference standard in the future.

Most diagnostic systematic reviews have examined the test performance characteristics of individual tests. While this is useful, we are often more interested in whether a new diagnostic test is better than current alternatives. Hence there is merit in designing systematic reviews to compare tests as the many biases and heterogeneity of results in primary studies are likely to be less important if tests are compared within individuals in each study.

8.2 Finding relevant studies

8.2.1 Finding existing systematic reviews

Appendix A gives information on finding existing systematic reviews. A check should be made of Database of Abstracts and Reviews (DARE) databases (available in the Cochrane Library or on the Internet) and MEDLINE. The DARE database compiles both intervention and diagnostic reviews, but not the other question types discussed in this guide. Even if the review is not considered completely appropriate, its reference list will provide a useful starting point.

8.2.2 Finding published primary studies

Initial searching should be done on MEDLINE, EMBASE and similar computerized databases. In MEDLINE, MeSH headings should be:

- the disease of interest (all subheadings), e.g.
  explode urinary tract infections
- the name of the test (all subheadings), e.g.
  explode reagent strips
- both the disease and the test, e.g.
  explode urinary tract infection AND explode reagent strips

Ideally, no further keywords should be used to restrict the search.

Only if inspection of the abstracts suggests that this initial approach is unmanageably nonspecific should the search be restricted. If you really need to restrict the search, try linking the disease and/or test (all subheadings) with the following:

> **sensitivity AND specificity** (exploded MeSH heading, which includes 'predictive value of tests' and 'receiver–operator (ROC) curve')
>
> OR
>
> **sensitivit*** (textword)
>
> OR
>
> **specificit*** (textword)
>
> OR
>
> **predictive value** (textword)

(Note: sensitivit* is a shorthand which allows for both 'sensitivity' and 'sensitivities').

This method of restricting the search while minimizing loss of sensitivity is based on evidence from a set of journals on general and internal medicine with high impact factors in 1986 and 1991 (Haynes et al., 1994). It may not be applicable now or to a wider range of journals. If it does not capture articles of known relevance, reconsider the feasibility of manually searching the abstracts of the unrestricted search based only on the disease and test. If you still consider that is not feasible, check how missed articles have been indexed to get ideas on additional restriction terms. Having two searchers develop strategies independently may be helpful. Some additional MeSH headings that may help generate relevant articles are:

diagnostic errors (exploded heading, which includes 'false-negative reactions', 'false-positive reactions' and 'observer variation')
diagnosis, differential
reproducibility of results
Some additional textwords that may help are:

accuracy, ROC, likelihood ratio

You may also find more articles by clicking on 'related articles' in relevant articles identified in PubMed (www.ncbi.nlm.nih.gov/Pub-Med/).

An alternative but perhaps less successful method of restricting is to search for the disease and/or test of interest, including only those subheadings concerned with diagnosis, for example:

diagnosis, pathology, radiography, radionuclide imaging, ultra-sonography and diagnostic use

Avoid using the MeSH heading 'diagnosis' because it differs from diagnosis as a subheading of a disease and is not designed to capture articles on diagnostic tests.

Articles on diagnostic tests may not be indexed as well as articles on intervention studies. Therefore, as demonstrated by the example of near-patient testing described in Section 2.3, it is more important to search the references of studies, handsearch relevant journals and conference proceedings and examine articles suggested by experts in the relevant field (McManus et al., 1998). It is helpful to record and report the details of your search strategy for future reference.

8.2.3 Finding unpublished primary studies

Publication bias is probably as much of a problem for systematic reviews of diagnostic tests as it is for observational studies in general. This is because reviews are often produced using available data sets and only those that show features of interest may reach publication.

Methods for detecting and dealing with publication bias for diagnostic test studies are not well developed. We are not aware of any attempt to develop registries of studies at the design stage, in the way that has been done for randomized controlled trials (RCTs).

8.3 Appraising and selecting studies

8.3.1 Standardizing the appraisal

The quality of diagnostic studies is determined by the extent to which biases have been avoided. However, a high-quality study (sometimes referred to as internally valid) may not be applicable in your setting (i.e. externally valid) if the exact test used differs from the one to which you have local access or the test has been evaluated in a tertiary care setting, while you are interested in using it in primary care. The applicability of high-quality studies is determined by whether the test methods and population accord with your area of interest.

Information about the characteristics that define the quality and applicability of studies may be used to decide the boundaries of the question to be answered by the systematic review, when reviewing abstracts or after having reviewed full papers. Alternatively, a more informative approach is to explore the extent to which some or all of the characteristics affect estimates of test performance when combining studies, as outlined in Section 8.4. For example, if the primary studies choose two different reference standards, it is possible to explore whether the estimated test performance characteristics vary with the choice of reference standard.

What study features should we assess?

Several checklists for quality and applicability of primary studies of diagnostic tests have been developed (Irwig et al., 1994; Jaeschke et al., 1994a,b; Reid et al., 1995; Liddle et al., 1996; Bruns, 1997). The most comprehensive checklist has been developed by the Cochrane Methods Working Group on Screening and Diagnostic Tests (www.cochrane.org/cochrane/sadt.htm). A shortened and updated version of this checklist is shown in Box 8.1. However, only a few studies are known that have given empirical evidence about the effect of quality on estimated test performance characteristics (Fahey et al., 1995; Lijmer et al., 1999). Nevertheless, any checklist should include the elements of quality and applicability outlined below.

Quality

1. Has selection bias been minimized?

   Consecutive patients with the features of interest should be enrolled. Some studies, however, do not use this method and instead estimate test performance based on people who have been diagnosed with the disease and those without the disease. These studies tend to include the more severe or definite end of the disease spectrum and the nondiseased group tends to be people without a clinical problem. Such 'case-control' studies are likely to overestimate both sensitivity and specificity (Lijmer et al., 1999).

2. Have adequate adjustments been made for residual confounding?

   For diagnostic tests, the issue of confounding can generally be considered as the incremental value of the new test over other tests that have been done (and which may be cheaper, less invasive, etc.). In this instance, this is an issue of applicability rather than quality and is discussed in more detail under applicability, below. Another context in which confounding arises is if the reference standard is a later event that the test aims to predict. In this case, any interventions should be blind to the test result, to avoid the 'treatment paradox': a test may appear to be poorly predictive because effective treatment in the test-positives has prevented the poor outcomes that the test would otherwise predict.

3. Have the final outcomes been adequately ascertained?

   To maintain the sample, all those enrolled should be verified by the reference standard and included in the analysis. Verification bias occurs when the reference standard is applied differently to the test-positives and the test-negatives. This is most likely when the reference standard is an invasive procedure, in which case the test-negatives are less likely to be subjected to it.

   Likewise, the proportion of the study group with unobtainable test results should be reported, for example the number of needle biopsies that provided an inadequate sample. It is inappropriate to omit from analysis those test results that are uncertain, for example

> The quality of reporting of diagnostic studies is often poor, making appraisal difficult

some, but not full-colour, development on a reagent strip. The test performance characteristics of uncertain test results should be obtained or uncertain results combined with positives or negatives.

4. Has measurement or misclassification bias been minimized?

A validated reference standard should be used and the test and reference standard should be measured independently of (blind to) each other. The tests should also be measured independently of other clinical and test information. Although independent assessment is generally desirable, there are some situations where prior information is needed, for example in identifying the exact site of an abnormality for which a radiograph is being viewed.

If tests are being compared, have they been assessed independently?

If tests are being compared, a systematic review based on studies in which the tests are being compared is a much stronger design than if performance characteristics of the tests come from different studies. The strongest within-study design is when both tests are done on the same individuals or individuals are randomly allocated to each test. It is especially important that two or more tests whose performance characteristics are being compared are assessed independently in each individual. For example, if mammography and ultrasound are being compared as a diagnostic aid in young women presenting with breast lumps, the two techniques should be assessed without knowledge of the results of the other imaging technique.

Applicability

Estimated test performance characteristics may depend heavily on details of how the test was performed and the population tested. This information should be collected and presented so that readers can judge applicability by the extent to which the clinical problem is being addressed and the exact test used is similar to those in the setting in which they practise.

About the test(s)
- How were tests performed (e.g. kits from different manufacturers)?

Box 8.1 Checklist for appraising the quality of studies of diagnostic accuracy

Descriptive information about the study
• Study identification
• What is the study type?
• What tests are being evaluated?
• What are the characteristics of the population and study setting?
• Is the incremental value of the test being compared to other routine tests?

Have selection biases been minimized?
• Were patients selected consecutively?

Have final outcomes been adequately ascertained?
• Is the decision to perform the reference standard independent of the test results (i.e. avoidance of verification bias)?
• If not, what per cent were not verified?

Have measurement biases been minimized?
• Was there a valid reference standard?
• Are the test and reference standards measured independently (i.e. blind to each other)?
• Are tests measured independently of other clinical and test information?
• If tests are being compared, have they been assessed independently (blind to each other) in the same patients or done in randomly allocated patients?

Has confounding been avoided?
• If the reference standard is a later event that the test aims to predict, is any intervention decision blind to the test result?

(modified from Cochrane Methods Working Group on Diagnostic and Screening Tests)

• What threshold was used to differentiate 'positive' from 'negative' tests?

  Ideally, tests will be looked at using several categories of test result (or even as a continuum), and this should be noted when it is done.

Because data are usually dichotomized around a single threshold in primary studies published to date, and accessible meta-analysis methods are best developed for dichotomized data, this will be the only approach considered further.

About the population
- Presenting clinical problem – the condition that defined entry into the study.
- Disease spectrum – the spectrum of disease in the diseased group (those with the disease of interest) is described directly by the stage or severity of disease. Spectrum in the so-called nondiseased group (those without the disease of interest) is described by the final diagnoses in that group. Indirect measures of spectrum include the setting (e.g. primary or tertiary care), previous tests and the referral filter through which people had to pass to get to the point where they were eligible for the study.
- Incremental value of tests – although a test may appear to give good results, it may not provide any more information than simpler (e.g. less invasive or cheaper) tests that are usually done in a particular setting. This is like thinking of these other tests as 'confounders' that must be taken into account when assessing the test performance characteristics of the test of interest (e.g. by restriction, stratification or modelling).

Indirect measures

The above features may not capture all aspects of quality and applicability, as the information you want is often not provided in the primary studies. Therefore, it is worth looking at some additional measures.
- Prevalence of the condition – this may be a proxy for the 'setting' in which the test is being assessed. More importantly, it has been shown that error in the reference standard is an important cause of sensitivity and specificity variation (nonlinear) with the observed prevalence of the condition (Brenner and Savitz, 1990; Valenstein, 1990).
- Year of the study – the quality of studies, the way tests have been done and the populations on which the tests are being performed may have altered over time.

Table 8.1. *Example summary table of quality features of a set of hypothetical diagnostic accuracy trials*

	Study descriptors				Quality	
Study	N	Setting	Consecutive attenders	Verification bias avoided	Test and reference standard measured independently	Tests being compared assessed independently
1	300	Hospital	Yes	Yes	Yes	Yes
2	800	Primary care	Yes	No	Yes	No
3	1000	Specialist clinic	No	Yes	No	Yes

8.4 Summarizing and synthesizing the studies

8.4.1 Presenting the results of the studies

Summary table

Studies should be listed, tabulating the extent to which they fulfil each criterion for quality and applicability (Table 8.1). Studies can be categorized by the most important quality and applicability criteria for the topic being addressed. If the number of studies is large or many criteria are considered equally important, provide a summary table showing the proportion of papers that fall into each category (or important combinations of criteria).

Graphical presentation

Simple plot of sensitivity and specificity
Show the sensitivity and specificity of each study with its confidence intervals. This is best done graphically, with the specificity for a particular study shown alongside the sensitivity for that study (as shown in Figure 8.1). Ordering the studies by some relevant characteristic helps interpretation. For example, test threshold may differ between studies, so that those studies with lowest sensitivity may have the highest specificity and vice versa. If studies are ranked by their specificity, the

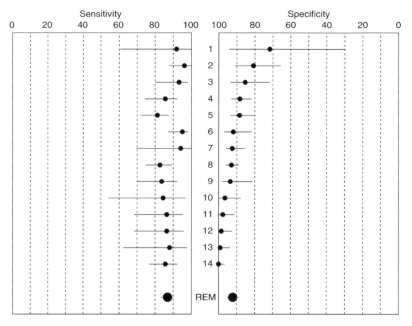

Figure 8.1   Plot of sensitivity versus specificity (with 95% confidence intervals) for 14 studies of carotid ultrasound for carotid stenosis (graph prepared with MetaTest software). REM, pooled estimate using the random effects model. Note that, as specificity improves, sensitivity appears to decrease. Data from Hasselblad and Hedges (1995).

visual display is the first step towards understanding the magnitude of this phenomenon.

The plot and all the following steps can be done using MetaTest software (see Appendix B). However, the currently available version of the software (MetaTest 0.5) does not test statistical significance. The Internet website will be updated as the software is developed further. Statistical modelling and significance testing can be done in any statistical package, but require expertise in applying the transformations outlined below and the back-transformation.

Plot sensitivity against specificity
The next step is to plot sensitivity against specificity in ROC space, ideally showing the points as ovoids with an area proportional to the square root of the number of people on whom sensitivity and specificity

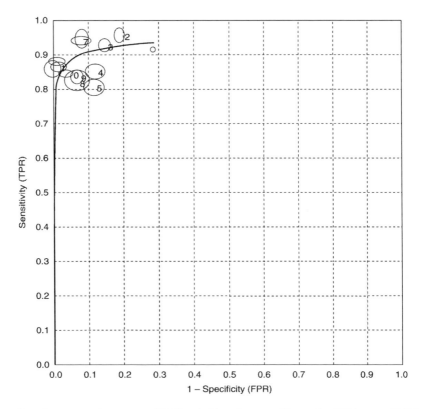

Figure 8.2   Receiver–operator curve (ROC) plotting true-positive rate (TPR: sensitivity) against false-positive rate (FPR: 1−specificity) for a meta-analysis of carotid ultrasound accuracy showing the individual study points and the fitted summary ROC (SROC). Data from Hasselblad and Hedges (1995).

have been calculated (Figure 8.2). As in the last step, this may display the tradeoff between sensitivity and specificity because studies have different thresholds.

8.4.2 Synthesis of study results

Fit a summary ROC (SROC)

A good method of combining data, which takes account of the interdependence of sensitivity and specificity, is the SROC (Moses et al., 1993; Irwig et al., 1994, 1995). This is difficult to do directly and is therefore done in three steps:

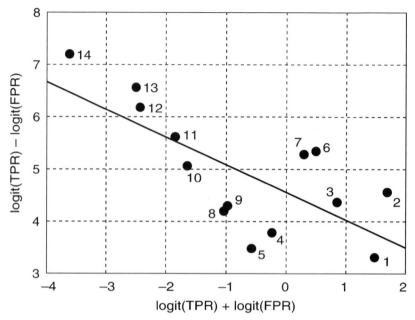

Figure 8.3

Plot of *D* versus *S* for a meta-analysis of carotid ultrasound accuracy showing the individual study points and the fitted line. Solid line shows unweighted best fit with intercept $a = 4.55$; slope $b = -0.53$. See text for details.

1. the true-positive rate (TPR, or sensitivity) and the false-positive rate (FPR, or 1 − specificity) are first transformed through the logarithm of their odds (a so-called 'logit' transformation);
2. the regression analysis is done; and
3. the results are back-transformed and plotted in the standard ROC format.

The transformation of the data in the second step examines the linear relationship:

$$D = a + bS$$

where: $D = (\text{logit TPR}) - (\text{logit FPR}) = \log (\text{odds ratio})$; $S = (\text{logit TPR}) + (\text{logit FPR})$ which is a proxy for the threshold; $a = $ estimated linear intercept; and $b = $ estimated regression coefficient (slope).

This relationship can be plotted as a regression of *D* on *S*, as shown in Figure 8.3, and provides the estimates of *a* and *b* needed for the SROC (Figure 8.2). If the slope, *b*, is nonsignificant and close to 0, then we can focus on the intercept, *a*, back-transforming it to the odds ratio. A single constant odds ratio defines a single symmetric SROC. If the slope, *b*, is significant, the situation is more complex – the odds ratio changes with the threshold, resulting in an asymmetric SROC.

One difficulty with SROC curves is that they do not give a particular set of sensitivity and specificity values as the summary estimate. We therefore suggest using the sensitivity at average specificity. For screening tests, read off the sensitivity at a false-positive rate (1 – specificity) equivalent to the positivity rate in your population. The sensitivity and specificity obtained can be used to generate post-test probabilities for a range of pretest values.

Compare tests

If the objective is to compare tests, use only those studies that do both tests and plot them using different symbols against the common SROC (Loy et al., 1996). Testing can be done by adding test type to the regression of the *D* (log odds ratio) on *S* (log odds product) mentioned in the previous section.

8.4.3 Assessing heterogeneity

Assess whether the test performance characteristics vary by study quality or population and test characteristics (Moons et al., 1997). Start by plotting the data for subgroups defined by each important criterion for study quality given in Section 8.3.1 and examine how they fall around the common regression. To test significance, add each feature individually in the SROC model. If there are sufficient studies, this can be extended to include several variables simultaneously using conventional approaches to modelling.

Questions for Part 2: diagnostic tests

1. Should positron emission tomography (PET) be used for the detection of mediastinal metastases in patients with lung cancer? You serve on a committee that is considering what uses of PET are warranted. One of the studies circulated for consideration at the

next meeting is the following paper: Dwamena, B., Sonnad, S., Angobaldo, J. and Wahl, R. (1999). Metastases from non-small cell lung cancer: mediastinal staging in the 1990s – meta-analytic comparison of PET and CT. *Radiology*, **213**, 530–6, which is also available on the web through: http://radiology.rsnajnls.org/.

(a) What are the strengths and weaknesses of this paper? Do you accept their conclusion?

(b) Are there any additional analyses which you would like to see on the data from the primary studies?

2. You decide to assess the quality of some of the primary studies yourself and select that by Steinert et al. on the grounds that this is one of the largest studies and had independent reading of computed tomography (CT) and PET according to Dwamena's meta-analysis. You find an abstract of the article by searching for the author's name on the journal website at: http://radiology.rsnajnls.org/search.dtl, and find an abstract which does not give you sufficient information about the study to allow you to appraise it. However, the website gives a list of other articles that cite the one by Steinert. One of them is: Kernstine, K. H., Stanford, W., Mullan, B. F. et al. (1999). PET, CT, and MRI with Combidex for mediastinal staging in non-small cell lung carcinoma. *Annals of Thoracic Surgery*, **68**, 1022–8. This covers the topic of interest to you and looks like it compares CT and PET. It is not mentioned in Dwamena and you presume it has been published since the search for studies for their review. You decide to assess its quality to decide whether it adds anything further to the results of Dwamena's review. You click on it and the website (http://ats.ctsnetjournals.org/cgi/content/full/68/3/1022) gives you the full text.

   • To what extent do you think the article fulfils the design criteria for primary studies?

   • Can you extract data to estimate the sensitivity and specificity of the tests if you wished to update the existing meta-analysis?

3. You decide the best evidence comes from head-to-head comparisons, including only those studies that compared PET and CT on the same patients.

   The data for this are not given directly in Dwamena's meta-analysis but can be worked out as the numbers of patients in each study and prevalence of metastases are given in Table 1 and the sensitivity and specificity in Table 2. Use MetaTest (see Appendix B) to analyse these data. On the basis of your analysis:

- What estimates of diagnostic odds ratio do you get for PET and CT?
- In how many of the studies is the diagnostic odds ratio higher for PET than for CT?
- Do the overall results suggest a conclusion different to that in Dwamena's meta-analysis?
- What is your overall conclusion?

Aetiology and risk factors

9.1 The question

Questions of aetiology and risk factors commonly arise in relation to public health. For example:

- Does the evidence support a likely causal effect of a factor (e.g. obesity) on a particular disease (e.g. breast cancer)?

Clearly, in public health terms, you may want to know the whole array of health effects of an exposure, but the evidence for each causal or preventive influence has to be first assessed separately, along the lines we suggest here. Largely, such evidence will come from case-control and cohort studies, although in some instances randomized controlled trials (RCTs) provide critical tests of causal hypotheses.

In a striking recent example, RCTs showed β-carotene to be an ineffective preventive of lung cancer, contrary to deductions made from a large number of observational studies that evaluated diet and laboratory data. This role of RCTs needs to be borne in mind when constructing a search strategy, as indicated below.

Getting the right balance in the question being addressed may be straightforward (e.g. 'Do oral contraceptives cause breast cancer?'), especially when it derives from a clear clinical or public health question. But should a review of body size and breast cancer include:

- all measures of body size (height, weight, skinfolds, circumferences, derived variables);
- only those that are modifiable (removing height, which is of biological interest); or
- only the most direct estimates of adiposity, such as skinfolds?

Such issues usually make systematic reviews of aetiology and risk factors more complex than systematic reviews of interventions.

9.1.1 Study design

Epidemiological studies of aetiology (often called observational studies) treat individual characteristics, personal behaviours, environmental conditions and treatments as 'exposures' that may modify risk of disease. In contrast with randomized trials, most epidemiological studies relate naturally occurring exposures to the onset of disease. These studies may be cross-sectional, prospective or retrospective. Cohort (prospective) studies relate exposure to subsequent onset of disease, comparing the rates among the exposed to that in the unexposed. Case-control studies compare the exposure histories of a group of cases to that among controls (disease-free).

> Cohort studies, which are similar in structure to a randomized trial, will generally provide the best aetiological studies

For the study of aetiology, good prospective studies often provide stronger evidence than case-control studies. Rarely are cross-sectional studies of importance, although in the case of obesity and breast cancer they may shed light on the relation between adiposity and hormone levels, giving support for a biological mechanism for the relation under study.

9.2 Finding relevant studies

9.2.1 Finding existing systematic reviews

You should first check whether an appropriate systematic review already exists (see Appendix A). If no such review is found or if none directly matches your needs and is up-to-date, then you face the challenge of constructing your own.

9.2.2 Finding published primary studies

The initial approach parallels that for searching for diagnostic studies, essentially searching MEDLINE for combinations of the disease, the exposure of interest and, if the resulting set is too large, adding a methodological filter. For example:

obesity AND breast cancer

will be quite specific, especially if combined with

human
OR
epidemiology

but much relevant research will be excluded, whereas

obesity OR any of its alternatives OR breast cancer

will spread a wider (more sensitive) net, but at the expense of retrieving a mass of unwanted material to sift through.

The amount of unwanted material can be reduced substantially by using a methodological filter, e.g. focusing on study types most likely to yield sound data relevant to causality, and/or pertinent measures of association (odds ratio, relative risk or hazard ratio).

It needs to be noted that, as with our suggestion above, the 'aetiological filter' excludes RCTs. In light of the β-carotene example (see Section 9.1), if such methodological filters are to be used, then RCTs should be included as a specific design option (as outlined in Section 6.2).

Your choice of a sensitive or a specific initial strategy will depend on your purpose – a fully comprehensive review requires the former as a starting point – and perhaps the size of the available literature (if it is small, you should probably scan it all anyway). But if you simply want a reasonable array of sound, relevant studies you should pursue a more restrictive search strategy from the start.

Finally, a comprehensive review should include handsearching of current relevant journals and scanning bibliographies of retrieved articles.

9.2.3 Finding unpublished primary studies

Relevant databases should be searched for possible unpublished work, including the database of dissertation abstracts. A number of services provide access to this and similar databases of unpublished thesis work. One useful source is the International Agency for Research on

Cancer (IARC) Directory of Ongoing Research in Cancer Prevention (Sankaranarayanan et al., 1996). This directory is available on the Internet from the IARC site. (www-dep.iarc.fr/prevent.htm).

9.3 Appraising and selecting studies

9.3.1 Standardizing the appraisal

The question at hand is whether any selection, measurement bias or confounding is great enough to seriously distort the size (and bias qualitative interpretation) of the effect estimate. The importance of these errors will vary with study type and problems specific to the question at hand. For example, exposure measurement error will be minimal for a biochemical value studied prospectively, but may be more important for self-reported exercise habits in a case-control study.

What study features should we assess?

Individual studies can be reviewed against a set of methodological criteria, systematically applied within study types. There are many different checklists that give different weight to elements of the design and conduct of observational studies. Box 9.1 gives an example derived from Liddle et al. (1996), which is a thoughtful publication in this area. For an alternative scale, see www.lri.ca/programs/ceu/oxford.htm.

The problems of bias and their solutions are qualitatively similar for case-control studies as for RCTs, although exposure measurement is usually far more challenging, and accessing a sufficient proportion of an appropriate control group often provides difficulties for case-control studies.

A reviewer must give greatest weight to factors that are most problematic for the issue under scrutiny, and then consistently assess their likely role in each study. It is also essential to consider the practical consequences of error. If, for example, despite the gross misclassification of physical activity due to poor patient recall, a study shows an association with, say, lower risks of osteoporosis, then the true effect of exercise is actually likely to be much larger than that observed.

1. Has sampling bias been minimized?

   Sampling (selection and allocation) bias arises when noncomparable criteria have been used to enrol participants in a case-control investigation.

2. Have adequate adjustments been made for residual confounding?

   In an RCT, given a reasonable randomization process (and large enough sample size), confounding should not be an issue, whereas for observational research it is always a possible explanation for an effect. Exactly how to proceed is not clear and attempts to deal with confounding in case-control and cohort studies deserve close attention (Colditz et al., 1995). Studies that do not control for known strong confounders (e.g. cigarette smoking in an analysis of diet and throat cancer) are likely to be of little value. One approach that has been used is to document the range of covariates considered in each of the studies identified and use this information to assess qualitatively the magnitude of confounding observed across the studies at hand.

   Better-quality studies always address confounding openly and thoughtfully, although this could lead to different actions. For example, include all possible confounders in a model; or exclude from a model variables that are shown not to confound, either practically (no/small change in estimate) or theoretically (not associated with exposure or not a risk indicator for disease).

   There will also be areas where knowledge of risk factors (and hence confounders) is limited, leading some authors to 'control' for confounding, while others do not. Here, considering whether adjusted and crude estimates differ may help judge whether confounder control implies higher quality. And it should always be borne in mind that even careful statistical control of many known confounders may still leave unknown or unmeasured confounding. This seems especially likely to occur with self-selection of life habits (e.g, exercise, long-term use of pharmaceutical preventives).

3. Have the final outcomes been adequately ascertained?

   In a prospective study, ascertainment bias arises when the intensity of surveillance and follow-up varies according to the exposure status of study participants. Documenting participation rates and methods of surveillance and diagnosis of endpoints is essential to assess sampling bias. Ascertainment bias may also arise when the actual diagnosis of interest is not independent of the exposure. This can arise in either prospective or retrospective studies.

4. Has measurement or misclassification bias been minimized?

Collection of noncomparable information from cases and non-cases accounts for measurement bias. This bias may arise when interviewers elicit information differentially between different study groups. Alternatively, participants may recall information with different levels of accuracy depending on their past disease experience. In retrospective or case-control studies this is referred to as recall bias.

> Quality is generally more difficult to achieve and to assess in observational studies than in randomized trials, but the issues are similar

Finally, measurement error due to general inaccuracy in the assessment of exposure leads to bias in the measure of association between exposure and outcome. In any study, if such error in exposure assessment is random, it will usually lead to underestimates of the association between exposure and disease.

9.4 Summarizing and synthesizing the studies

9.4.1 Presenting the results of the studies

Summary table

A summary table is essential to show individual study characteristics. You should prepare a common data abstraction form on to which to summarize the main elements of each study:

- descriptive data on numbers, demographic and other characteristics; and
- relevant outcome measures – frequencies, effect estimates (simple, adjusted, ordered) and confidence intervals or P values, in particular.

And be warned – this abstract form should be extensively piloted before starting the summary table itself. It can be hard to imagine the array of different ways results of observational studies are presented. Early consultation with a statistician may also be helpful in deciding how to deal with (and record) an absence of point estimates and/or confidence intervals, and factors that are sometimes treated as a cause (e.g. overweight) and elsewhere as preventive (e.g. low/normal weight). Analyses over a range of doses will also often be based on different categories in different settings.

Here and elsewhere in the presentation of results, it is best to begin by considering studies according to study design. That is, evaluate the prospective studies as a group and compare the results with those reported from the case-control studies, and from any RCTs. Such presentation sets the stage for combining data within each study design type as a first step in data summarization.

Graphical presentation

The best way to show the pattern of effects is to plot point estimates (generally shown with 95% confidence intervals). There should be some sensible order to the data, for example, ranking or grouping by quality score or study type, and examining them for consistency (or lack thereof) first within and then across groups. Whether or not it is sensible or useful to combine the estimates across all studies, or sub-groups, is a decision to be made, as noted previously, according to subjective judgements (perhaps aided by a formal test of heterogeneity) on the data pattern and the similarity of the studies.

9.4.2 Synthesis of study results

The estimates in observational studies will usually need to be adjusted for the major confounding factors such as age, gender, etc. A quantitative synthesis will thus aim at combining these adjusted estimates. Hence, the methods described in Section 6.4 (Interventions) will only occasionally be applicable. However, the general principle will still be to obtain a weighted combination where the weights are the inverse of the variance of the estimator. Thus, the standard error of each adjusted estimate will be required. If this is not given directly, it may need to be inferred from the confidence interval (the width of which will be about 4 standard errors of the log risk ratio or odds ratio on a log scale) or the exact P value. Several software packages now automate these calculations for use in meta-analysis.

Box 9.1 Checklist for appraising the quality of studies of risk factors and aetiology

This set of criteria should be used for appraising studies of the extent to which the characteristics or behaviour of a person, an environmental exposure or the characteristics of a disease alter the risk of an outcome.

Information about the study Description
- Study identification
- What is the study type?
- What risk factors are considered?
- What outcomes are considered?
- What other factors could affect the outcome(s)?
- What are the characteristics of the population and study setting?

Evaluation criteria for the study
Criterion fulfilled
- Are study participants well-defined in terms of time, place and personal characteristics?
- What percentage of individuals or clusters refused to participate?
- Are outcomes measured in a standard, valid and reliable way?
- Are risk factors and outcomes measured independently (blind) of each other?
- Are all important risk factors included in the analysis?
- What percentage of individuals or clusters recruited into the study are not included in the analysis (i.e. lost to follow-up)?
Overall assessment of the study
- How well does the study minimize bias? What is the likely direction in which bias might affect the study results?
- Include other comments concerning areas for further research, applicability of evidence to target population, importance of study to policy development.

Source: modified from Liddle et al. (1996).

Ideally, all studies should have been adjusted for all major confounders. If some have not, then these would need to be grouped separately, or external adjustments made. A good general discussion of such methods for synthesis of observational studies is available in Rothman and Greenland (1998; see the chapter on meta-analysis).

9.4.3 Assessing heterogeneity

Heterogeneity arises when the results vary among the studies more than can be attributed to chance (see Section 4.3). The 'homogeneity assumption' is that the results of all studies estimate the same true effect and that the observed variation is due to within-study sampling error. However, in practical research applications it is impossible to know whether this is true, and it is most likely that it is not.

Many investigators use statistical tests of heterogeneity (lack of homogeneity) to see whether the assumption is correct, and to evaluate the test at the $P = 0.05$ level (see Section 4.3). However, because these tests have low power, homogeneity should not be assumed uncritically. That is, the purpose of the test is not to determine whether heterogeneity exists at all, but to get an idea of how much heterogeneity exists.

For observational studies there are more sources of heterogeneity than for RCTs. For example, where a series of RCTs may have all used the same doses of a drug and a common protocol for definition of the endpoint of interest, there is relatively little potential for variation among the studies. For observational studies, however, the approach to measuring the exposure may vary among the studies, and the criteria used for diagnosis or the class of endpoints studied often also differ. When the intensity of surveillance for endpoints differs across studies, there is a range of sources of heterogeneity.

Therefore, for observational studies, in particular, it is better to act as if there is heterogeneity among study results when the χ^2 goodness-of-fit test statistic is greater than the number of studies minus 1 (which is the mean value when there is no heterogeneity).

If the purpose of meta-analysis is to study a broad issue then the true values can be expected to vary from study to study, and both an estimate of this variability and the mean of the true values are important and should be reported (Colditz et al., 1995). The contribution of factors such as study design and methods to the observed heterogeneity can then be evaluated.

9.5 Judging causality

Once the most important features of the data and the heterogeneity between studies have been explored with respect to study-specific flaws of sample (size and/or selection bias), measurement or confounding, the reviewer is positioned to explore formally whether the observed effects allow a causal interpretation.

- Is there a clear (reasonably strong) and important effect, which is fairly consistently seen, at least among the better studies?
- Has the effect been demonstrated in human experiments?
- Is this effect greater at higher exposures?
- Does it have an accepted or probable biological basis?
- Is it evident that the time direction of the association is clear (cause always precedes effect)?

Other elements may be added, such as those suggested by Bradford Hill (1965). Studies that provide a critical test of a causal hypothesis are particularly important. These will often be experimental studies, as with the β-carotene example described in Section 9.1. However you approach it, there is no doubt that a careful and logical assessment of the broad causal picture is extremely helpful to a reader struggling to understand the mass of facts a review may contain.

> There is no easy formula for judging causality, which is based on the strength and consistency of multiple evidence

Questions for Part 2: aetiology and risk

1. You are sitting on a prevention advisory panel for your state department of public health. The committee is charged with updating prevention recommendations for women's cancers. You are asked to make recommendations for ovarian cancer. A colleague suggests that, based on the meta-analysis by Hankinson, you should recommend that all women take oral contraceptives for at least 5 years to halve their risk of ovarian cancer. You wonder what the evidence is for this and track down the Hankinson paper (see abstract below).

Obstetrics and Gynecology (1992). **80,** 708–14.

A quantitative assessment of oral contraceptive use and risk of ovarian cancer

Hankinson SE, Colditz GA, Hunter DJ, Spencer TL, Rosner B, Stampfer MJ

Channing Laboratory, Department of Medicine, Harvard Medical School, Boston, Massachusetts.

OBJECTIVE: To provide a quantitative assessment of the association between oral contraceptive (OC) use and ovarian cancer using results from the published literature. DATA SOURCES: We conducted a MEDLINE literature search for all epidemiologic studies of OC and ovarian cancer published in English between 1970–1991. The reference list for each article was reviewed to locate additional published articles. METHODS OF STUDY SELECTION: We included 20 studies in which a relative risk and either a standard error, confidence interval, or *P* value was reported, or sufficient data were presented to allow us to calculate these measures. DATA EXTRACTION AND SYNTHESIS: We summarized the findings using weighted averages and regression analyses. We found a summary relative risk of 0.64 (95% confidence interval 0.57–0.73) associated with eve-use of OC, indicating a 36% reduction in ovarian cancer risk. The risk of ovarian cancer decreased with increasing duration of OC use; we noted a 10–12% decrease in risk with 1 year of use and approximately a 50% decrease after 5 years of use. The reduced risk was present among both nulliparous and parous women and it appeared to last for at least 10 years after cessation of use. Although most studies assessed the use of OC formulations from the 1960s and 1970s, data from the Cancer and Steroid Hormone Study indicate that the decreased ovarian cancer risk may also be present with current lower-dose formulations. CONCLUSION: The protective effect of OC against ovarian cancer risk should be considered in a woman's decision to use OC.

Before accepting the conclusions, you decide that it is worth checking that the authors did a good job of the review and, in particular, you decide to look at whether they did a thorough literature search, to check that the studies were of adequate quality, and verify whether they did an acceptable job of combining the studies, including looking at differences between studies and possible heterogeneity.

(a) Read the meta-analysis of oral contraceptives and risk of ovarian cancer and assess for yourself whether the methods were valid.

(b) What issues arise out of the meta-analysis and what further questions might the authors address?

(c) What are the implications for prevention recommendations from this meta-analysis?

2. Read two of the studies – the Walnut Creek study and the CASH study – and see whether you agree with the meta-analysts' conclusions about the quality (see checklist in Box 9.1) and data from these studies.

3. Using the data in the Hankinson paper (see the CD), try to replicate the analysis of the authors. (You might use the 'metareg' macro in Stata to do the analysis.)

Prediction: prognosis and risk

10.1 The question

Prognostic questions generally contain two parts:
- the definition of the patient population of interest, e.g. recent-onset diabetes, newly detected colorectal cancer; and
- the outcomes of interest, such as morbidity and mortality.

The implicit third part of the usual three-part question is the set of risk factors that have been used for the prediction of prognosis. Chapter 9 looked at a single risk factor, with a particular focus on whether that risk factor was causally associated with the outcome. In this chapter this idea is extended but with a focus on prediction or prognosis for individuals. This chapter should therefore be read in conjunction with Chapter 9 on risk factors but differs in two ways.
- Firstly, the principal aim is prediction of outcomes, whether or not the factors are causal. For example, an earlobe crease might be considered a valid marker of cardiovascular disease risk and form a useful part of a risk prediction model, though clearly it is a marker rather than being causal.

Prediction of risk is important for assessing who will benefit most from treatment

- Secondly, the combination of multiple factors for prediction will often give better prediction than the single factors considered in Chapter 9 (e.g. Framingham cohort study risk equations for heart disease).

10.1.1 Why should we be interested in prediction?

There are two principal reasons for investigating questions about prediction. Firstly, patients are intrinsically interested in their prognosis, so that they can adapt and plan for their future. Secondly, separation of individuals with the same disease into those at high and low risk may be extremely valuable in appropriately targeting therapy. Generally, those with high risk have more to gain, and hence benefits are more likely to outweigh disadvantages, and also to be more cost-effective.

In using prognostic information to help decide on treatment, it is generally important to know the natural history of the condition. That is, what would happen without any effective therapy? It is important to realize that this is often impossible information to collect, as some therapy will often have been started. Hence it is important to consider that prognosis is conditional. For example, you may ask about the prognosis of noninsulin-dependent diabetic patients conditional on antihypertensive treatment being given for high blood pressure and antihypercholesterolaemic agents being given for high cholesterol levels.

The placebo groups of trials may be considered a reasonable source of information for natural history but even these groups will often be undergoing some forms of treatment and the new treatment that is being compared with placebo is as an add-on to these other therapies.

10.1.2 Study design

The ideal study design for prognostic studies should focus on cohort studies with an inception cohort of patients with a condition followed for a sufficiently long period of time for the major outcomes to have occurred.

10.2 Finding relevant studies

10.2.1 Finding existing systematic reviews

Systematic reviews for the influence of single factors on prognosis are becoming more common (e.g. the effect of blood pressure level on stroke risk) and it is clearly worth trying to find them using the methods described in Part 1 and Appendix A. However, there are methodological problems for systematic reviews that look at several prognostic factors simultaneously and hence only a few have been undertaken.

10.2.2 Finding published primary studies

The search strategies given in Appendix A (Haynes et al., 1994) focus on identifying longitudinal studies that potentially have such predictive information. An important alternative to consider is the use of the control groups in randomized controlled trials (RCTs), as this is often the only place where sufficient investment in follow-up has been made to be able to provide adequate information on prognosis.

10.2.3 Finding unpublished primary studies

Since there is no registry of prognostic studies, these will be particularly difficult to track down. Some exceptions occur when routine data are kept on a group of patients. For example, cancer registries provide locally relevant survival data, although the degree of detail on prognostic factors varies considerably.

10.3 Appraising and selecting studies

10.3.1 Standardizing the appraisal

What study features should we assess?

The requirements for good-quality information on prognosis are similar to those of an RCT (see Section 6.3). The two principal differences are that randomization is unnecessary, but that good baseline measurements of the potential prognostic factors have been included. The following information is critical to appraise.

1. Has selection assignment bias been minimized?

    A consecutive or random sample of patients should have been selected at a similar time point in their disease. If this is at the beginning of the disease, this is known as an 'inception cohort'.

2. Have adequate adjustments been made for residual confounding?

    Confounding plays a very different role when we are focused on risk prediction rather than aetiology. Even if confounders are not causal, but merely good markers of risk, they may be useful in a prognostic or prediction model. Hence they do not need to be used for adjustment but may be a useful part of the model. However, if the population used to develop the model differs importantly from the target population then an adjustment for this difference would be needed (e.g. if the populations differed in age or gender).

3. Have final outcomes been adequately ascertained?

Having obtained a representative group through consecutive or random selection, high rates of follow-up and inclusion of all patients are important. Hence, it is desirable to extract and report data on the level of follow-up.

4. Has measurement or misclassification bias been minimized?

Outcomes should preferably be measured blind to the prognostic factors being considered. For example, knowing about factors such as cholesterol or smoking may influence the decision about whether a person has ischaemic heart disease. This becomes more common if the outcome to be assessed is more subjective and hence more open to observer bias.

10.4 Summarizing and synthesizing the studies

10.4.1 Presenting the results of the studies

A summary table of the identified studies should be included with both the characteristics of the study population, the follow-up and outcomes measured, and the quality features mentioned in the previous section.

In this case the data must be emphasized because multiple factors and synthesis across several studies are usually much more difficult or even impossible to deal with. Hence, it may be necessary to forgo any synthesis, and choose the largest acceptable quality study available.

It should be noted, however, that the study with the largest number of patients will not necessarily be the most statistically reliable. It is the outcomes that really provide the information, and this will depend on three factors:

• the number of patients;
• the length of follow-up; and
• the level of risk of the patients.

The number of patients and the length of follow-up combined represent the total 'person time' of the study, which is commonly used as a measure of the relative power of studies.

10.4.2 Synthesis of the studies

Combining studies is occasionally possible, although it is uncommon. Ideally, this would involve the use of individual patient data pooled from the studies. One example of this is the INDANA project, which has pooled the prognostic information from several trials of hypertension (Gueffier et al., 1995). Another example is the Atrial Fibrillation Trialists Collaborative, which has combined prognostic information on patients with atrial fibrillation (Atrial Fibrillation Investigators, 1994).

However, as discussed in Part 1, combining studies is sometimes impossible and, even if it is possible, it requires considerable effort and cooperation. It also relies on common prognostic factors having been measured at a baseline, and in a similar way. For example, the atrial fibrillation collaboration could not include the predictive value of echocardiograms because most studies had not included this as a prognostic measure. Hence, such pooling will usually be confined to the prognostic factors common to all studies.

> Combining studies with multiple risk predictors is complex and usually not possible

(Statistical note: it may not be necessary to combine all of the individual data in a single file but may be sufficient to pool the variance–covariance matrices – see the *Handbook of Research Synthesis*, Cooper and Hedges 1994.)

10.4.3 Assessing heterogeneity

When considering single prognostic factors, the issues and methods are similar to those for intervention studies (see Section 6.4.3). That is, is there heterogeneity of the size of the effect, and is it explained by study design or patient factors? However, for multiple-factor prognostic studies, appropriate methods have not been described. If there is a pooling of individual study data then each factor within the multivariate model could be examined to check whether there were interactions with other factors.

Appendixes

Literature searching

This appendix contains further advice about searching: firstly, some general tips; secondly, finding existing systematic reviews; thirdly, finding randomized trials; and fourthly, using methodological filters.

Finding existing systematic reviews

As discussed in Chapter 1, it is always worth checking to see whether a systematic review or meta-analysis has already been done. Even if it needs modification or updating, it will provide a useful base of studies and issues. For interventions, Cochrane reviews are available in the Cochrane Database of Systematic Reviews (CDSR) in the Cochrane Library, which also contains the Database of Abstracts and Reviews (DARE) database. The DARE database compiles and appraises many nonCochrane reviews of both interventions and diagnostic accuracy.

Several different strategies have been developed for identifying systematic reviews in electronic databases. For example, Hunt and McKibbon (1997) have developed simple and complex search strategies for MEDLINE for finding systematic reviews and meta-analyses, which are applicable to all question types.

Some alternative strategies (Boynton et al., 1998) are available at the York Centre for Reviews and Dissemination.

A simple search strategy (high precision, low sensitivity) is:
MEDLINE [ab]
Comment [pt]
Letter [pt]
Editorial [pt]

General tips for searching (from McKibbon et al., 1999)

1. Use multiple bibliographic databases (MEDLINE, CINAHL, EMBASE/Excerpta Medica, and psycINFO will cover most of the mainstream health care literature).
2. Use databases of different kinds (e.g. citation, theses, research, PubMed related articles feature).
3. Extend the years of searching.
4. Have more than one set of searchers do your main searching independently – each searcher will retrieve relevant, unique citations.
5. Find out how the articles that you already have are indexed and work backwards using the index terms from the original article. Bibliographies and personal files are often good places to find relevant citations to start with.
6. Avoid major emphasis (starring).
7. Avoid, or use AND NOT carefully. You can NOT out what you are truly interested in.
8. Avoid subheadings – use other methods of limiting information.
9. Make sure you are using all the explodes that are possible AND make sense.
10. Make sure you know the definitions of the terms you are using, e.g. in MEDLINE adults are anyone who is from 19 to 44 years old – anyone over the age of 45 is considered to be middle-aged.
11. Remember the specificity rule in constructing strategies (e.g. definition of 'nutrition' may need many terms or groupings of terms (vitamin deficiency, protein restriction, and so on)).
12. Use a combination of textwords and index words.
13. For textwords make sure you remember: alternative spellings (randomized and randomised); differences in terminology across disciplines (bed sores and decubitus ulcers); terminology across national boundaries (SIDS and cot death); differences in historical naming (unwed mothers, *Campylobacter pylori*); short forms for terms (AIDS and acquired immunodeficiency syndrome); brand and generic names (Viagra and sildenafil).
14. Make sure you use terms that are somewhat related (mortality and survival analysis).
15. Use author searching, study names (GISSI, GUSTO, SOLVD), locations (Mayo Clinic), manufacturers of drugs or products.
16. Search using opposites for some topics (e.g. if you are interested in 'tallness' make sure you search for 'being short' too).

Golden rule of searching
Keep track of what you have done!

A more comprehensive search strategy is to combine (AND) the following:

Meta[ab]

synthesis [ab]

literature [ab]

randomized [hw]

published [ab]

meta-analysis [pt]

extraction [ab]

trials [hw]

controlled [hw]

MEDLINE [ab]

selection [ab]

sources [ab]

trials [ab]

review [ab]

articles [ab]

reviewed [ab]

english [ab]

language [ab]

comment [pt]

letter [pt]

editorial [pt]

Finding randomized trials

The following search strategy (developed by Kay Dickersin) is used by the Cochrane Collaboration to identify randomized trials in MEDLINE. This search is run regularly and forms part of the process of identifying trials for the Cochrane Controlled Trials Registry.

#1 RANDOMIZED-CONTROLLED-TRIAL in PT

#2 CONTROLLED-CLINICAL-TRIAL in PT

#3 RANDOMIZED-CONTROLLED-TRIALS

#4 RANDOM-ALLOCATION

#5 DOUBLE-BLIND-METHOD

#6 SINGLE-BLIND-METHOD

#7   #1 or #2 or #3 or #4 or #5 or #6
#8   TG = ANIMAL not (TG = HUMAN and TG = ANIMAL)
#9   #7 not #8
#10 CLINICAL-TRIAL in PT
#11 explode CLINICAL-TRIALS
#12 (clin* near trial*) in TI
#13 (clin* near trial*) in AB
#14 (singl* or doubl* or trebl* or tripl*) near (blind* or mask*)
#15 (#14 in TI) or (#14 in AB)
#16 PLACEBOS
#17 placebo* in TI
#18 placebo* in AB
#19 random* in TI
#20 random* in AB
#21 RESEARCH-DESIGN
#22 #10 or #11 or #12 or #13or #15 or #16 or #17 or #18 or #19 or
     #20 or #21
#23 TG=ANIMAL not (TG=HUMAN and TG=ANIMAL)
#24 #22 not #23
#25 #24 not #9
#26 TG=COMPARATIVE-STUDY
#27 explode EVALUATION-STUDIES
#28 FOLLOW-UP-STUDIES
#29 PROSPECTIVE-STUDIES
#30 control*or prospectiv* or volunteer*
#31 (#30 in TI) or (#30 in AB)
#32 #26 or #27 or #28 or #29 or #31
#33 TG=ANIMAL not (TG=HUMAN and TG=ANIMAL)
#34 #32 not #33
#35 #34 not (#9 or #25)
#36 #9 or #25 or #35

PubMed clinical queries using research methodology filters

A free MEDLINE facility is available from the National Library of
Medicine (www.nlm.nih.gov/). A section of this is the PubMed Clinical

Table A1. *Clinical queries using research methodology filters*

Category	Optimized for:	ELHILL terms[a]	Sensitivity/specificity[b]	PubMed equivalent[c]
Therapy	Sensitivity	Randomized controlled trial (pt) or drug therapy (sh) or therapeutic use (sh) or all random: (tw)	99%/74%	'randomized controlled trial' [PTYP]	'drug therapy' [SH]	'therapeutic use' [SH:NOEXP]	'random*' [WORD]
	Specificity	All double and all blind: (tw) or all placebo: (tw)	57%/97%	(double [WORD] & blind* [WORD])	placebo [WORD]
Diagnosis	Sensitivity	Exp sensitivity a#d specificity or all sensitivity (tw) or diagnosis & (px) or diagnostic use (sh) or all specificity (tw)	92%/73%	'sensitivity and specificity' [MESH]	'sensitivity' [WORD]	('diagnosis' [SH]	'diagnostic use' [SH]	'specificity' [WORD]
	Specificity	Exp sensitivity a#d specificity or all predictive and all value: (tw)	55%/98%	'sensitivity and specificity' [MESH]	('predictive' [WORD] & 'value*' [WORD]
Aetiology	Sensitivity	Exp cohort studies or exp risk or all odds and all ratio: (tw) or all relative and all risk (tw) or all case and all control: (tw)	82%/70%	'cohort studies' [MESH]	'risk' [MESH]	('odds' [WORD] & 'ratio*' [WORD])	('relative' [WORD] & 'risk' [WORD])	('case' [WORD] & 'control*' [WORD])
	Specificity	Case-control studies or cohort studies	40%/98%	'case-control studies' [MH:NOEXP]	'cohort studies' [MH:NOEXP]
Prognosis	Sensitivity	Incidence or exp mortality or follow-up studies or mortality (sh) or all prognos: (tw) or all predict: (tw) or all course (tw)	92%/73%	'incidence' [MESH]	'mortality' [MESH]	'follow-up studies' [MESH]	'mortality' [SH]	prognos* [WORD]	predict* [WORD]	course [WORD]
	Specificity	Prognosis or survival analysis	49%/97%	prognosis [MH:NOEXP]	'survival analysis' [MH:NOEXP]

[a] MEDLINE terms used by ELHILL (search engine for MEDLARS and Grateful MED).

[b] Sensitivity, the proportion of high-quality studies in MEDLINE that are detected, specificity, the proportion of irrelevant or poorer-quality studies detected.

[c] Approximate equivalent in PubMed query language, as used on the Clinical Queries Using Research Methodology Filters page (www.ncbi.nlm.nuh.gov/entrez/query.fcgi).

Queries, which uses methodological filters developed by Haynes et al. (1994) for many of the question types discussed in Part 2 of this book. These searches, which are shown in Table A1, are less extensive than the methods discussed in Part 2, but may be useful as a quick initial search.

Software for meta-analysis

Many standard statistical software packages provide facilities that would facilitate meta-analysis (e.g. by the use of logistic regression). Some packages have had routines or macros specifically developed to allow meta-analysis. For example, STATA has a macro for the analysis of multiple 2×2 table data (this is available in the *STATA Technical Bulletin Reprints*, 7, sbe16: Meta-analysis. S. Sharp & J. Sterne, www.stata.com).

In addition to standard statistical software, over the last several years a number of programs specifically designed to perform meta-analysis have been developed, some of which are described below. None of these is comprehensive or capable of performing all of the types of analysis discussed in Part 2. In particular, there is only one program available for performing adequate meta-analytic studies. Even for a single question type, however, it may be necessary to use more than one package to achieve an adequate range of analyses. Some of the packages are freely available and others are commercial packages costing a few hundred dollars. This list is not comprehensive; another listing is also available on the Internet (www.bmj.com/cgi/content/full/316/7126/221).

Meta-analysis of intervention study

RevMan

This is the standard systematic review software for the Cochrane Collaboration (hiru.mcmaster.ca/cochrane/). This is a comprehensive package for managing the process of systematic reviews of intervention studies. RevMan is used for the writing of protocols, keeping the list of included and excluded publications, writing the Cochrane Review Text and performing the statistical meta-analytic functions. This last task is done through a separate program – MetaView – which then enables the final reviews published in the Cochrane Library to be analysed by the same piece of software. Because of its comprehensive nature and structured processes, the package can be slightly more difficult to learn than most others. RevMan 4.1 was released in 2000.

MetaAnalyst

This is an MS-DOS program developed by Dr Joseph Lau at the New England Medical Center and New England Cochrane Center in the United States. MetaAnalyst is designed to analyse a set of trials; the data from each trial can be presented as a 2×2 table. The program performs a wide variety of meta-analytic statistics on trial data, providing both fixed and random fixed models for relative risk, odds ratio and risk differences. It also provides heterogeneity statistics, cumulative meta-analytic plots and regressions against control rate, all with publication-quality plots; however, the types of print are limited.

EasyMA

EasyMA is an MS-DOS program with a user-friendly interface developed to help physicians and medical researchers to synthesize evidence in clinical or therapeutic research. The program was developed by the Michel Cucherat, a teaching hospital in Lyon, France. The latest version (98c) is available on the Internet (www.spc.univ-lyon.fr/~mcu/easyma/).

SCHARP

The Survival Curve and Hazard Ratio Program (SCHARP) for meta-analysis of individual patient data was developed by the Medical Research Council Cancer Trials Office, Cambridge, UK and the Instituto Maria Negri, Milan, Italy. This is a Windows-based menu-driven program aimed at producing summary survival plots and forest plots of the hazard ratios. It is planned that SCHARP should be made freely available in 1999.

Comprehensive Meta-analysis

This is a versatile Windows 95/98/2000 program. Like RevMan, it creates a database of studies, with full citations which can be imported from MEDLINE. Data may be entered in a wide variety of formats, with conversions performed automatically. The available effect size indices include mean difference, correlations, rate difference, relative risk and odds ratio with both fixed and random effects models. The graphs allow subgroup, and cumulative meta-analyses with publication-quality graphs. Additional graphs include funnel plots. Data can be directly entered or imported from Excel (www.Metaanalysis.com).

Meta-analysis of diagnostic tests

MetaTest

This is an MS-DOS program developed by Dr Joseph Lau at the New England Medical Center and New England Cochrane Center in the United States. This is the only available software package which produces a comprehensive meta-analysis of diagnostic test accuracies. The plots include simple plots of sensitivity and specificity with their confidence intervals, summary receiver–operator curve (ROC) plots giving the data points of the individual studies, and a summary ROC (see Chapter 8). It is available on the Internet (www.cochrane.org/cochrane/sadt.htm).

MetAxis

This program is produced by Update Software, who also produce RevMan for the Cochrane Collaboration. It is aimed at the whole systematic review process, not just the meta-analytic calculations. It will include methods for interventions studies and diagnostic studies. For details, see www.update-software.com/metaxis.

Glossary

Absolute risk reduction (risk difference)

>The effect of a treatment can be expressed as the difference between relevant outcomes in treatment and control groups by subtracting one rate (given by the proportion who experienced the event of interest) from the other. The reciprocal is the number needed to treat (NNT).

Accuracy (*see also* validity)

>The degree to which a measurement represents the true value of the variable which is being measured.

Adverse event

>A nonbeneficial outcome measured in a study of an intervention that may or may not have been caused by the intervention.

Allocation (or assignment to groups in an intervention study)

>The way that subjects are assigned to the different groups in an intervention study (e.g. drug treatment/placebo; usual treatment/no treatment). This may be by a random method (*see* randomized controlled trial) or a nonrandom method.

Applicability (*see also* external validity, generalizability)

>The application of results to both individual patients and groups of patients. This term is preferred to generalizability as it includes the idea of particularizing or individualizing treatment and is closest to the general aim of clinical practice. It addresses whether a particular treatment that showed an overall benefit in a study might be expected to convey the same benefit to an individual patient.

Before-and-after study (*see also* pretest–post-test study)

>A study design where a group of subjects is studied before and after an intervention. Interpretation of the result is problematic as it is difficult to separate the effect of the intervention from the effect of other factors.

Bias

>Bias is a systematic deviation of a measurement from the 'true' value, leading to

either an over- or underestimation of the treatment effect. Bias can originate from many different sources, such as allocation of patients, measurement, interpretation, publication and review of data.

Blinding

Blinding or masking is the process used in epidemiological studies and clinical trials in which the observers and the subjects have no knowledge as to which treatments subjects are assigned. This is done in order to minimize bias occurring in patient response and outcome measurement. In single-blind studies only the subjects are blind to their allocations, whilst in double-blind studies both observers and subjects are ignorant of the treatment allocations.

Bradford Hill criteria (*see* causality)

Case-control study

Patients with a certain outcome or disease are selected together with an appropriate group of controls without the outcome or disease. The groups are then compared with the populations which have been exposed to the factor under investigation.

Case series

The intervention has been used in a series of patients (it may or may not be a consecutive series) and the results reported. There is no separate control group for comparison.

Causality

The relating of causes to the effects they produce. The Bradford Hill criteria for causal association are temporal relationship (exposure always precedes the outcome – the only essential criterion), consistency, strength, specificity, dose–response relationship, biological plausibility, coherence and experiment.

Clinical outcome

An outcome for a study that is defined on the basis of the disease being studied (e.g. fracture in osteoporosis, peptic ulcer healing and relapse rates).

Clinically important effect (*see also* statistically significant effect)

An outcome that improves the clinical outlook for the patient. The recommendations made in clinical practice guidelines should be both highly statistically significant and clinically important (so that the 95% confidence interval includes clinically important effects).

Cochrane Collaboration

The Cochrane Collaboration is an international network that aims to prepare, maintain and disseminate high-quality systematic reviews based on randomized controlled trials (RCTs) and when RCTs are not available, the best available evidence from other sources. It promotes the use of explicit methods to minimize bias, and rigorous peer review.

Cohort study

Groups who have been exposed, or not exposed, to a new technology or factor of interest are followed forward in time and their rates of developing disease (or achieving cure, etc.) are compared.

Comparative study

A study including a comparison or control group.

Concurrent controls

Controls receive the alternative intervention and undergo assessment concurrently with the group receiving the new intervention. Allocation to the intervention or control is generally not random when this term is used.

Confidence interval

An interval within which the population parameter (the 'true' value) is expected to lie with a given degree of certainty (e.g. 95%).

Confounding

The measure of a treatment effect is distorted because of differences in variables between the treatment and control groups that are also related to the outcome. For example, if the treatment (or new intervention) is trialled in younger patients then it may appear to be more effective than the comparator, not because it is better, but because the younger patients had better outcomes.

Cross-sectional study

Also called prevalence study, where both exposure and outcomes are measured at the same time.

Cumulative meta-analysis

In a systematic review, the results of the relevant studies are ordered by some characteristic and sequential pooling of the trials is undertaken in increasing or decreasing order.

Degrees of freedom (df)

The number of independent comparisons that can be made between the members of a sample.

Double-blind study (*see* blinding)

Ecological fallacy

The bias that may occur because an association observed between variables on an aggregate (e.g. country) level does not necessarily represent the association that exists at an individual (subject) level.

Effectiveness

The extent to which an intervention produces favourable outcomes under usual or everyday conditions.

Effect modification, effect modifier (*see also* interaction)

The relationship between a single variable (or covariate) and the treatment effect. Significant interaction between the treatment and such a variable indicates that the treatment effect varies across levels of this variable.

Efficacy

The extent to which an intervention produces favourable outcomes under ideally controlled conditions such as in a randomized controlled trial.

Efficiency (technical and allocative)

The extent to which the maximum possible benefit is achieved out of available resources.

Evidence-based medicine/health care

The process of finding the best relevant research information in the medical literature to address a specific clinical problem. This evidence is then combined with clinical expertise and the patient values in making individual decisions.

External validity (*see also* generalizability, applicability)

Also called generalizability or applicability, this is the degree to which the results of a study can be applied to situations other than those under consideration by the study, for example, for routine clinical practice.

Extrapolation

This refers to the application of results to a wider population and means to infer, predict, extend or project the results beyond that which was recorded, observed or experienced.

Generalizability (*see also* external validity, applicability)

This refers to the extent to which a study's results provide a correct basis for generalization beyond the setting of the study and the particular people studied. It implies the application of the results of a study to another group or population.

Gold standard

A method, procedure or measurement that is widely regarded or accepted as being the best available. Often used to compare with new methods.

Hazard ratio (HR)

When time to the outcome of interest is known, this is the ratio of the hazards in the treatment and control groups where the hazard is the probability of having the outcome at time t, given that the outcome has not occurred up to time t.

Heterogeneity

This refers to the differences in treatment effect between studies contributing to a meta-analysis. If there is significant heterogeneity, this suggests that the trials are not estimating a single common treatment effect.

Historical controls

Data from either a previously published series or treated patients previously at an institution are used for comparison with a prospectively collected group of patients exposed to the technology or intervention of interest at the same institution.

Incidence

The number of new events (new cases of a disease) in a defined population, within a specified period of time.

Intention to treat

An analysis of a clinical trial where participants are analysed according to the group to which they were initially randomly allocated, regardless of whether or not they dropped out, fully complied with the treatment or crossed over and received the other treatment. By preserving the original groups one can be more confident that they are comparable.

Interaction (*see* effect modification)

The relationship between a single variable (or covariate) and the treatment effect.

Interrupted time series

Treatment effect is assessed by comparing the pattern of (multiple) pretest scores and (multiple) post-test scores (after the introduction of the intervention) in a group of patients. This design can be strengthened by the addition of a control group which is observed at the same points in time but the intervention is not introduced to that group. This type of study can also use multiple time series with staggered introduction of the intervention.

Intervention

An intervention will generally be a therapeutic procedure such as treatment with a pharmaceutical agent, surgery, a dietary supplement, a dietary change or psychotherapy. Some other interventions are less obvious, such as early detection (screening), patient educational materials or legislation. The key characteristic is that a person or his or her environment is manipulated in the hope of benefiting that person.

Level of evidence

Study designs are often grouped into a hierarchy according to their validity, or degree to which they are not susceptible to bias. The hierarchy indicates which studies should be given most weight in an evaluation.

Magnitude of treatment effect

This refers to the size of the summary measure (or point estimate) of the treatment effect. This may be absolute (*see* absolute risk reduction and number needed to treat) or relative (*see* relative risk).

Meta-analysis

Results from several studies, identified in a systematic review, are combined and summarized quantitatively.

Meta-regression

The fitting of a linear regression model with an estimate of the treatment effect as the dependent variable and study level descriptors as the independent variables.

Nonrandomized cross-over design

Participants in a trial are measured before and after introduction or withdrawal of the intervention and the order of introduction and withdrawal is not randomized.

Number needed to harm (NNH)

When the treatment increases the risk of the outcome, then the inverse of the absolute risk increase is called the number needed to harm (NNH).

Number needed to treat (NNT)

NNT is the number of patients with a particular condition who must receive a treatment for a prescribed period in order to prevent the occurrence of specified adverse outcomes of the condition. This number is the inverse of the absolute risk reduction.

Observational studies

Any nonrandomised, nonexperimental comparison.

Odds ratio (OR)

Ratio of the odds of the outcome in the treatment group to the corresponding odds in the control group. For low risk, this is usually very similar to the relative risk.

Patient's expected event rate (PEER)

> The probability that a patient will experience a particular event (e.g. a stroke or myocardial infarction) if left untreated. Also known as baseline risk or absolute risk without treatment.

Patient-relevant outcome

> Any health outcome that is meaningful to the patient. It can be the best surrogate outcome, resources provided as part of treatment, impact on productivity (indirect) or one that cannot be measured accurately (e.g. pain, suffering). Common examples include: primary clinical outcomes, quality of life and economic outcomes.

Pretest–post-test study

> Outcomes (pain, symptoms, etc.) are measured in study participants before they receive the intervention being studied and the same outcomes are measured after. 'Improvement' in the outcome is reported. Often referred to as before-and-after studies.

Prevalence

> The measure of the proportion of people in a population who have some attribute or disease at a given point in time or during some time period.

Prognostic model

> A statistical model that estimates a person's probability of developing the disease or outcome of interest from the values of various characteristics (such as age, gender, risk factors).

Publication bias

> Bias caused by the results of a trial being more likely to be published if a statistically significant benefit of treatment is found.

P value (*see also* confidence interval, statistically significant effect)

> The probability that the null hypothesis (that there is no treatment effect) is incorrectly rejected.

Quality of evidence

> Degree to which bias has been prevented through the design and conduct of research from which evidence is derived.

Quality of life

> The degree to which a person perceives him or herself able to function physically, emotionally and socially. In a more quantitative sense, an estimate of remaining life free of impairment, disability or handicap as captured by the concept of quality-adjusted life years (QALYs).

Random error

The portion of variation in a measurement that has no apparent connection to any other measurement or variable, generally regarded as due to chance.

Randomization

A process of allocating participants to treatment or control groups within a controlled trial by using a random mechanism, such as coin toss, random number table or computer-generated random numbers.

Randomized controlled trial

An experimental comparison study in which participants are allocated to treatment/intervention or control/placebo groups using a random mechanism (*see* randomization). Participants have an equal chance of being allocated to an intervention or control group and therefore allocation bias is minimized (and virtually eliminated in very large studies).

Randomized cross-over trial

Patients are measured before and after exposure to different interventions (or placebo) which are administered in a random order (and usually blinded).

Relative risk or risk ratio (RR)

Ratio of the proportions in the treatment and control groups with the outcome. This expresses the risk of the outcome in the treatment group relative to that in the control group.

Relative risk reduction (RRR)

The relative reduction in risk associated with an intervention. This measure is used when the outcome of interest is an adverse event and the intervention reduces the risk. It is calculated as one minus the relative risk, or:

RRR = 1 − (event rate in treatment group/event rate in control group)

Reliability

Also called consistency or reproducibility. The degree of stability that exists when a measurement is repeatedly made under different conditions or by different observers.

Risk difference (RD)

The difference (absolute) in the proportions with the outcome between the treatment and control groups. If the outcome represents an adverse event (such as death) and the risk difference is negative (below 0) this suggests that the treatment reduces the risk – referred to as the absolute risk reduction.

Selection bias

Error due to systematic differences in characteristics between those who are selected for study and those who are not. It invalidates conclusions that might otherwise be drawn from such studies.

Statistically significant effect (*see also* clinically important effect)

An outcome for which the difference between the intervention and control groups is statistically significant (i.e. the P value is ≤ 0.05). A statistically significant effect is not necessarily clinically important.

Strength of evidence

Magnitude, precision and reproducibility of the intervention effect (including magnitude of the effect size, confidence interval width, P value and the exclusion of clinically unimportant effects). In the case of nonrandomized studies, additional factors such as biological plausibility, biological gradient and temporality of associations may be considered.

Surrogate outcome

Physiological or biochemical markers that can be relatively quickly and easily measured and that are taken as predictive of important clinical outcomes. They are often used when observation of clinical outcomes requires longer follow-up. (Also called intermediate outcomes.)

Systematic review

The process of systematically locating, appraising and synthesizing evidence from scientific studies in order to obtain a reliable overview.

Time series

A set of measurements taken over time. An interrupted time series is generated when a set of measurements is taken before the introduction of an intervention (or some other change in the system), followed by another set of measurements taken over time after the change.

Validity

- Of measurement: an expression of the degree to which a measurement measures what it purports to measure; it includes construct and content validity.
- Of study: the degree to which the inferences drawn from the study are warranted when account is taken of the study methods, the representativeness of the study sample and the nature of the population from which it is drawn (internal and external validity, applicability, generalizability).

Acronyms and abbreviations

ACP	American College of Physicians
AIDS	acquired immune deficiency syndrome
CCTR	Cochrane Controlled Trials Registry
CD-ROM	compact disk-read only memory
CDSR	Cochrane Database of Systematic Reviews
CI	confidence interval
Cochran Q	Cochran χ^2
DARE	Database of Abstracts and Reviews (Cochrane Library)
ECG	electrocardiogram
exp	explode
FPR	false-positive rate
GP	general practitioner
HIV	human immunodeficiency virus
HR	hazard ratio
IARC	International Agency for Cancer Research
MeSH	Medical Subject Heading
NHMRC	National Health and Medical Research Council
NLM	National Library of Medicine (United States)
NNH	number needed to harm
NNT	number needed to treat
OR	odds ratio
P	probability
PEER	patient's expected event rates
RCT	randomized controlled trial
RD	risk difference
ROC	receiver–operator curve
RR	relative risk or risk ratio
SCHARP	Survival Curve and Hazard Ratio Program, developed by MRC Cancer Trials Office, Cambridge, UK
SROC	summary receiver–operator curve
TPR	true-positive rate

References

Allen, I.E. and Olkin, I. (1999). Estimating time to conduct a meta-analysis from number of citations retrieved. *Journal of the American Medical Association*, **282**, 634–5.

Atrial Fibrillation Investigators (1994). Risk factors for stroke and efficacy of antithrombotic therapy in atrial fibrillation: pooled data from five randomised controlled trials. *Archives of Internal Medicine*, **28**, 957–60.

Begg, C.B. and Mazumdar, M. (1994). Operating characteristics of a rank correlation test for publication bias. *Biometrics*, **50**, 1088–101.

Berlin, J. (1997). Does binding of readers affect the results of meta-analyses? *Lancet*, **350**, 185–6.

Boynton, J., Glanville, J., McDaid, D. and Lafabvre, C. (1998). Identifying systematic review in MEDLINE: developing an objective approach to search strategy design. *Journal of Information Science*, **24**, 137–57.

Bradford Hill, A. (1965). The environment and disease: association or causation. *Proceedings of the Royal Society of Medicine*, **58**, 295–300.

Brenner, H.S. and Savitz, D.A. (1990). The effects of sensitivity and specificity of case selection on validity, sample size, precision, and power in hospital-based case-control studies. *American Journal of Epidemiology*, **132**, 181–92.

Breslow, N.E. and Day, N.E. (1987). *Statistical Methods in Cancer Research 2: The Design and Analysis of Cohort Studies*. Lyon: IARC.

Bruns, D.E. (1997). Reporting diagnostic accuracy. *Clinical Chemistry*, **43**, 2211.

Caldwell, M. and Watson, R. (1994). Peritoneal aspiration cytology as a diagnostic aid in acute appendicitis. *British Journal of Surgery*, **81**, 276–8.

Clarke, M. and Hopewell, S. (2000). Time lag bias in publishing results of clinical trials: a systematic review. In *Third Symposium on Systematic Reviews: Beyond the Basics*, p. 21. Oxford, United Kingdom: St Catherine's College.

Colditz, G.A., Burdick, E. and Mosteller, F. (1995). Heterogeneity in meta-analysis of data from epidemiologic studies: a commentary. *American Journal of Epidemiology*, **142**, 371–82.

Cooper, A.J. (1998). Systematic review of *Propionibacterium acnes* resistance to systemic antibiotics. *Medical Journal of Australia*, **169**, 259–61.

Cooper, H. and Hedges, L.V. (eds) (1994). *Handbook of Research Synthesis*. New York: Russell Sage Foundation.

Detsky, A., Naylor, C.D., O'Rourke, K., McGreer, A.J. and L'Abbe, K.A. (1992). Incorporating variations in the quality of individual randomized trials into meta-analysis. *Journal of Clinical Epidemiology*, **45**, 255–65.

Dickersin, K., Min, Y.I. and Meinert, C.L. (1992). Factors influencing publication of research results: followup of applications submitted to two institutional review boards. *Journal of the American Medical Association*, **267**, 374–8.

Drummond, M.F., O'Brien, B., Stoddart, G.L. and Torrance, G.W. (1997). *Methods for the Economic Evaluation of Health Care Programmes*. Oxford: Oxford University Press.

EBCTCG (Early Breast Cancer Trialists' Collaborative Group) (1992). Systematic treatment of early breast cancer by hormonal cytotoxic or immune therapy: 133 randomised trials involving 31 000 recurrences and 24 000 deaths among 75 000 women. *Lancet*, **339**, 71–85.

Egger, M., Smith, G.D., Schneider, M. and Minder, C. (1997). Bias in meta-analysis detected by a simple, graphical test. *British Medical Journal*, **315**, 629–34.

Fahey, M., Irwig, L. and Macaskill, P. (1995). Meta analysis of pap test accuracy. *American Journal of Epidemiology*, **141**, 680–9.

Gelber, R. and Goldhirsch, A. (1987). Interpretation of results from subset analyses within overviews of randomised clinical trials. *Statistics in Medicine*, **6**, 371–8.

Gueffier, F., Boutitie, F., Boissel, J.P. et al. (1995). INDANA: a meta-analysis on individual patient data in hypertension. Protocol and preliminary results. *Therapie*, **50**, 353–62.

Guyatt, G.H. and Rennie, D. (1993). User's guide to medical literature. *Journal of the American Medical Association*, **270**, 2096–7.

Guyatt, G.H., Sackett, D.L. and Cook, D.J. (1993). Users' guides to the medical literature. II. How to use an article about therapy or prevention. A. Are the results of the study valid? Evidence-Based Medicine Working Group. *Journal of the American Medical Association*, **270**, 2598–601.

Guyatt, G.H., Sackett, D.L. and Cook, D.J. (1994). Users' guides to the medical literature. II. How to use an article about therapy or prevention. B. What were the results and will they help me in caring for my patients? *Journal of the American Medical Association*, **271**, 59–63.

Hasselblad, V. and Hedges, L.V. (1995). Meta-analysis of screening and diagnostic tests. *Psychological Bulletin*, **117**, 167–78.

Haynes, R.B., Wilczynski, N., McKibbon, K.A., Walker, C.J. and Sinclair, J.C. (1994). Developing optimal search strategies for detecting clinically sound studies in Medline. *Journal of the American Medical Informatics Association*, **1**, 447–58.

Henry, D. (1992). Economic analysis as an aid to subsidisation decisions: the development of Australian guidelines for pharmaceuticals. *PharmacoEconomics*, **1**, 54–67.

Hunt, D.L. and McKibbon, K.A. (1997). Locating and appraising systematic reviews. *Annals of Internal Medicine*, **126**, 532–8. (http://www.acponline.org/journals/annals/01apr97/systemat.htm)

Irwig, L., Tosteson, A.N.A., Gastonis, C. et al. (1994). Guidelines for meta-analyses evaluation of diagnostic tests. *Annals of Internal Medicine*, **120**, 667–76.

Irwig, L., Macaskill, P., Glasziou, P. et al. (1995). Meta-analytic methods for diagnostic test accuracy. *Journal of Clinical Epidemiology*, **48**, 119–30.

Jackson, R. (2000). Updated New Zealand cardiovascular disease risk–benefit prediction guide. *British Medical Journal*, **320**, 709–10.

Jaeschke, R., Guyatt, G. and Sackett, D.L. (1994a). Users' guides to the medical literature. III. How to use an article about a diagnostic test. A. Are the results valid? *Journal of the American Medical Association*, **271**, 389–91.

Jaeschke, R., Guyatt, G.H. and Sackett, D.L. (1994b). Users' guides to the medical literature. III. How to use an article about a diagnostic test. B. What are the results and will they help me in caring for my patients? *Journal of the American Medical Association*, **271**, 703–7.

Juni, P., Witschi, A., Bloch, R. and Egger, M. (1999). The hazards of scoring the quality of clinical trials for meta-analysis. *Journal of the American Medical Association*, **208**, 1054–60.

L'Abbe, K.A., Detsky, A.S. and O'Rourke, K. (1987). Meta-analysis in clinical research. *Annals of Internal Medicine*, **107**, 224–33.

Liddle, J., Williamson, M. and Irwig, L. (1996). *Method for Evaluating Research and Guideline Evidence*. Sydney: NSW Health Department.

Lijmer, J., Mol, B., Heisterkamp, S., Bonsel, G.J. and Bossuyt, P. (1999). Empirical evidence of bias in the evaluation of diagnostic tests. *Journal of the American Medical Association*, **282**, 1061–6.

Linde, K., Ramirez, G., Mulrow, C.D. et al. (1996). St John's wort for depression – an overview and meta-analysis of randomised clinical trials. *British Medical Journal*, **313**, 253–8.

Loy, C.T., Irwig, L.M., Katelaris, P.H. and Talley, N.J. (1996). Do commercial serological kits for *Helicobacter pylori* infection differ in accuracy? A meta-analysis. *American Journal of Gastroenterology*, **91**, 1138–44.

Mahoney, M.J. (1977). Publications prejudices: an experimental study of confirmatory bias in the peer review system. *Cognitive Therapy and Research*, **1**, 61–75.

McKibbon, A., Eady, A. and Marks, S. (1999). *PDQ Evidence-based Principles and Practice*. B.C. Decker.

McManus, R.J., Wilson, S., Delaney, B.C. et al. (1998). Review of the usefulness of contacting other experts when conducting a literature search for systematic reviews. *British Medical Journal*, **317**, 1562–3.

Moons, K.G., van Es, G.A., Deckers, J.W., Habbema, J.D. and Grobbee, D.E. (1997). Limitations of sensitivity, specificity, likelihood ratio and Bayes' theorem in assessing diagnostic probabilities: a clinical example. *Epidemiology*, **8**, 12–17.

Moses, L., Shapiro, D. and Littenberg, B. (1993). Combining independent studies of a diagnostic test into a summary ROC curve: data analytic approaches and some additional considerations. *Statistics in Medicine*, **12**, 1293–316.

Mulrow, C.D. and Oxman, A. (1996). *How to Conduct a Cochrane Systematic Review*. 3. Oxford: The Cochrane Collaboration.

Mulrow, C.D. and Oxman, A. (1997). *Cochrane Collaboration Handbook* (updated Sept 1997). Oxford: The Cochrane Collaboration.

NHMRC (National Health and Medical Research Council) (1999a). *A Guide to the Development, Implementation and Evaluation of Clinical Practice Guidelines*. Canberra: NHMRC.

NHMRC (1999b). *How to Use the Evidence: Assessment and Application of Scientific Evidence*. Canberra: NHMRC.

NHMRC (1999c). *How to Assess the Costs: Evaluation of Economic Evidence*. Canberra: NHMRC.

Reid, M.C., Lachs, M.S. and Feinstein, A.R. (1995). Use of methodological standards in diagnostic test research. Getting better but still not good. *Journal of the American Medical Association*, **274**, 645–51.

Rosenthal, A. (1979). The file drawer problem and tolerance for null results. *Psychological Bulletin*, **86**, 638–41.

Rothman, K.J. and Greenland, S. (1998). *Modern Epidemiology*. Philadelphia: Lippincott–Raven.

Sankaranarayanan, R., Becker, N. and Demaret, E. (1996). *Directory of Ongoing Research in Cancer Epidemiology*. International Agency for Cancer Reseach (IARC) scientific publication no. 137. (see www-dep.iarc.fr/prevent.htm)

Schmid, C.H., McIntosh, M., Cappelleri, J.C., Lau, J. and Chalmers, T.C. (1995). Measuring the impact of the control rate in meta-analysis of clinical trials. *Controlled Clinical Trials*, **16**, 66s.

Schmid, C.H., Lau, J., McIntosh, M. and Cappelleri, J.C. (1998). An empirical study of the effect of the control rate as a predictor of treatment efficacy in meta-analysis of clinical trials. *Statistics in Medicine*, **17**, 1923–42.

Schulz, K.F., Chalmers, I., Hayes, R.J. et al. (1995). Empirical evidence of bias: dimensions of methodological quality associated with estimates of treatment effects in controlled trials. *Journal of the American Medical Association*, **273**, 408–12.

Self, P.C., Filardo, T.W. and Lancaster, F.W. (1989). Acquired immunodeficiency syndrome (AIDS) and the epidemic growth of its literature. *Scientometrics*, **17**, 49–60.

Sharp, S.J., Thompson, S.G. and Altman, D.G. (1996). The relation between treatment benefit and underlying risk in meta-analysis. *British Medical Journal*, **313**, 735–8.

Simes, R. (1987). Confronting publication bias: a cohort design for meta-analysis. *Statistics in Medicine*, **6**, 11–29.

Stern, J. and Simes, R.J. (1997). Publication bias: evidence of delayed publication in a cohort study of clinical research projects. *British Medical Journal*, **315**, 640–5.

Thompson, S.G. (1995). Why sources of heterogeneity in meta-analysis should be investigated. *British Medical Journal*, **309**, 1351–5.

Towler, B., Irwig, L., Glasziou, P. et al. (1998). A systematic review of the effects of screening for colorectal cancer using the faecal occult blood test, Hemoccult. *British Medical Journal*, **317**, 559–65.

Tramer, M.R., Reynolds, D.J.M., Moore, R.A. and McQuay, H.J. (1997). Impact of covert duplicate publication on meta-analysis: a case study. *British Medical Journal*, **315**, 635–40.

Valenstein, P.N. (1990). Evaluating diagnostic tests with imperfect standards. *American Journal of Clinical Pathology*, **93**, 252–8.

Walter, S.D. (1997). Assessing the relationship between effect size and baseline risk in the context of meta-analyses. *Statistics in Medicine*, **16**, 2883–900.

Whitehead, A. and Whitehead, J. (1991). A general parametric approach to the meta-analysis of randomized clinical trials. *Lancet*, **10**, 1665–77.

Index

Numbers in italics indicate *tables* or *figures*